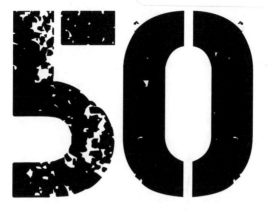

Fitness Tips

You <u>Wish</u> You Knew

Derek Doepker

ExcuseProof.com

Disclaimer:

Copyright 2012, All rights reserved.

Table of Contents

Preface:

- Do you know there's a brain "hack" that can stop emotional food cravings dead in their tracks that doesn't require superhuman willpower?

- Do you know what motivates every person on this planet can be boiled down to six basic human needs, and by understanding these you can *program* yourself to drop any bad habit and replace it with a better habit - even if you've constantly struggled before?

- Do you know the rarely talked about force stronger than willpower that will make or break your fitness success?

- Do you know there's a way to literally rewire your brain and reprogram your genetics so you can be more resistant to stress, live longer, and stay leaner?

- Do you know the majority of people who go on a diet and lose weight often gain it all back because they fail to do *this* one simple thing?

- Do you know the #1 thing holding people back from ideal health isn't a poor diet, lack of exercise, or even their genetics?

- Do you know there's a way to make raw spinach taste absolutely delicious, in under 60 seconds, *without* needing a blender, juicer, or any special kitchen equipment, and it works even if you normally *hate* the taste of leafy greens?

- Do you know there's a way to make healthy food from scratch that's easier, tastier, cheaper, and *faster* than fast food?

- Do you know why relying on a multi-vitamin is not enough to insure good health, and what you really need to make sure your body gets the nutrition it needs to burn fat, build muscle, and stay healthy?

- Do you know there's a type of (affordable) herb that will go into your body, and fix whatever *you* uniquely need fixed, all without harmful side effects?

- Do you know that if you shop at most major supplement retailers, you're paying 2-3 times as much as you need to for products that are lower quality than when you shop *here*?

- Do you know the truth about detoxing and how it can <u>really</u> be done safely and effectively?

These are just a handful of things *I wish I knew* back when I first got started. But instead of having all these secrets laid out for me in one valuable and easy to read guide, I spent the past nine years and thousands of hours of research digging through countless resources on health, exercise, advanced supplementation, psychology, herbalism, neuroscience, and more to figure all this stuff out.

But I didn't just study, I experimented on myself and sifted and sorted through all the stuff I read to separate fact from fiction. The problem usually isn't in finding information on weight loss, health, and fitness as I'll readily admit with enough research you can find plenty of good information for free on google or in the library. The problem is typically finding *too much* information and getting overwhelmed with conflicting advice. Google "fitness tips" and you can spend the rest of your life sorting through 319 million pages of information. Would you rather do that research yourself to separate what works from what is bogus, or let someone who's done the research for you (by spending thousands of hours and dollars learning from the world's best) hand you the "keys to the kingdom" in one simple and easy to read guide?

80-90% of the things in this book are things I've utilized myself to get and stay fit, overcome health challenges, and do so while on a busy schedule and limited budget. The other 10-20% comes from sources that I trust and are much smarter than I am in their respective fields. In truth, the majority of what I share can be traced back to pioneers who discovered it before I did, so I try my best to give credit to where credit is due.

A lot of books on health and fitness advice out there are simply rehashing old material without offering anything new and valuable. This rarely provides you, the reader, with something that is *cutting-edge* and truly worth spending your time and money on. While I can't promise every single thing in this guide will "blow your mind" or be something you didn't already know or couldn't find elsewhere with enough digging around, I can promise you I've really strived to create a fitness book unlike *anything* else you've ever read.

The truth is, the best ways to get fit and healthy usually aren't anything "new." You probably already know a lot of the common sense things that you can do to move towards your fitness goals. The real challenge is figuring out how to *actually apply* those things we all know we should do. I believe the best way I can assist you in doing that is by providing a new way of looking at things you may not have ever considered. This typically means providing insightful reasons *why* certain tips are so incredibly beneficial and/or *how* to make following a particular strategy to be in great shape that extra bit easier so you'll successfully stick with it.

Whether you wish you had more motivation, wish you had an easier time staying fit on a busy schedule or on a budget, or simply are someone like myself with a never ending curiosity for how to "hack" the body and mind, I've made it my mission to make this one of the most **valuable** books you will ever read for not only changing your body, but changing your entire life.

How To Use This Book

Tips 1-15 are centered around mindset and motivation, and I consider them must-reads for everyone as they reveal some of the most neglected but <u>essential</u> insights for not just getting fit and healthy, but also maintaining a **permanently** lean body for the rest of your life.

Tips 16-30 are centered around healthy eating. I consider them very useful for people who want to know how to spice up their diet, eat healthy in a hurry, and eat healthier on a limited budget. This isn't a book on what to eat or laying out a specific diet plan. You can find plenty of that stuff elsewhere. Instead, these tips will provide simple tricks to make following a healthier eating plan *much* easier.

For additional insights on motivation tips on healthy eating, I also have a book available called How To Stick To A Diet available in both print format and kindle format at: excuseproof.com/diet

Tips 31-40 are centered around natural health remedies and supplements. Not all of these tips will be applicable to everyone, so pick and choose what you feel is most beneficial to you without getting overwhelmed by all the various potential recommendations. I do my best to lay out what is merely helpful vs. "essential" for the average person.

Tips 41-50 are centered around exercise and training. These tend to be tips for exercising at home, on a limited budget, and with limited time. Many of these tips can be incorporated into an exercise routine one is already doing. I don't like to offer too much in the way of specific training programs as that is highly unique to individual's body type and goals, but I provide a few resources to where you can find more training programs for free online. A website like t-nation.com provides a variety of training programs primarily aimed at muscle and strength building, but there are programs equally as productive for fat loss and women's goals there as well. A home workout like P90X is suitable for many people's needs, but it is far from the only good home workout program. In the resources section, I share some one of my favorite training programs.

About The Author

My name is Derek Doepker I didn't always use to be the super healthy and motivated guy I am today. I started out as a 17 year old high school student who ate fast food *every single night*. I refused to eat healthy. I never exercised leaving me one of the most out of shape guys in my class.

I started to read about the effects an unhealthy lifestyle was having on the body and made a commitment to change. Even though I hated eating healthy foods and exercising, I discovered how to change my mindset and stick with with a healthy eating plan and exercise routine that allowed me to add over 30 pounds of muscle in several months, and get a ripped six pack in the process.

I then went on to help my overweight friend, Shane Edele, drop from 220 pounds to 168 pounds. He now maintains a six pack year round. We've both been able to maintain our physiques and healthy eating habits with ease over the course of 8 years since we've started thanks to many of the tips I'm going to share with you.

Today, I am a fitness author and founder of Excuse Proof Fitness at excuseproof.com. I wrote this book because I want to help others avoid all of the mistakes I've made, and give you the secrets I've picked up over the years for how to stay fit no matter what obstacles you face. I believe many of the things I'm going to share with you are absolutely life changing far beyond their effects on health and fitness.

These techniques are based on what has worked for me and many others, but don't just believe anything I say. Rather, try it for yourself and see what works for you. You may find these tips are simply a spring board for you to find your own unique solutions. And I myself am always updating and refining my recommendations as new research emerges. I certainly can be wrong about anything I write here, but I do my best to provide only the most proven and time tested strategies.

Just to let you know I practice what I preach, here is a picture of me that shows what I look like all year-round.

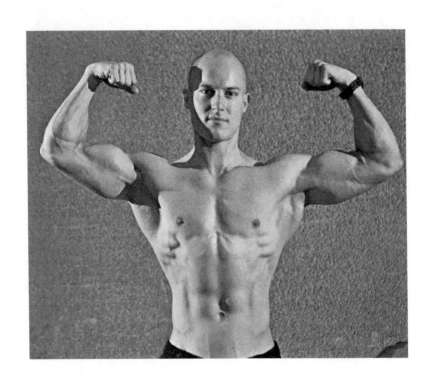

Free Gift

I'd like to reward you with free access to my premium fitness newsletter.

You'll learn my best cutting edge strategies for getting fit on a busy schedule, how to reprogram your genetics, and get "insider" tips picked up from the world's elite fitness trainers. Simply visit excuseproof.com and get free instant access to the Excuse Proof Fitness Survival Guide and newsletter today.

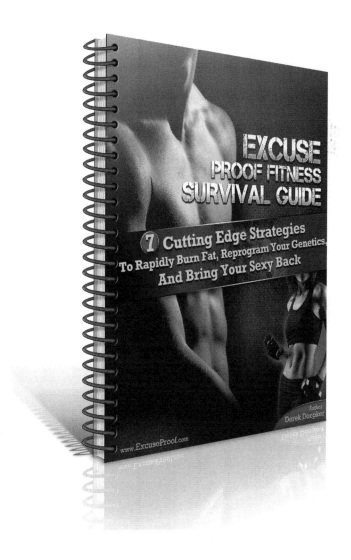

1: The Key To Permanent Weight Loss And Success

The promises of losing 30 pounds in 30 days offered by many fitness programs sure sound sexy, but they don't always address a very important detail – is that weight loss sustainable? What good does it do anyone to get fast results with weight loss, muscle gain, or improved health only to lose all of those results shortly after?

This is a sad reality as studies show a large portion of people who lose significant amounts of weight through dieting fail to keep it off over the long haul. But the problem isn't, as some people claim, purely because "diets don't work" or that obesity is a matter of genetic set-points. While there is some truth to the idea that short-term dietary quick-fixes typically don't work over the long haul, that's often because they leave out the most critical element to long term success.

Before I understood this critical element, I failed to see why some people like myself were able to maintain their fit physiques for many years straight while other people would constantly struggle with weight loss and weight regain often accompanied with yo-yo dieting efforts. Then I started studying psychology, personal development, and simply observed those who were successful and found it wasn't a genetic factor that was making a difference, it was a mental one.

That is, people who not only get results, but *keep* those results are those who've made health and fitness a **habitual lifestyle** rather than simply a means to an end. When healthy eating and exercise are your habits, the results they bring are both permanent and come with greater ease.

The challenge is that over 90% of your day to day actions are not conscious choices, but done out of habit. And simply consciously deciding to do something different like cut out junk food and eat healthier isn't always enough to overcome years of engrained eating and lifestyle habits. Particularly when one's habits have a strong emotional component. Hence, the New Year's Resolutions that never quite pan out by February.

Is there a solution?

Yes. And you don't even need to read the books on psychology and neuroscience like I have to figure out the practical methods of changing your habits. While many of the tips in this guide work together to help you change your habits, this tip is simply about the importance of taking gradual steps.

This method of changing your health habits is simple. Pick *only* 1 or 2 things a month that you want to change. They should be challenging, but something you know you will be able to do.

Examples include:

- Walking 10 minutes a day 3 times a week.

- Carrying a gallon of water with you at all times and drinking it regularly.

- Replacing 1 sugary drink with green tea each day.

- Doing a set of 20 pushups, body-weight squats, and resistance band rows after waking up.

The following month, either add in a new behavior you'd like to make a habit or simply add more effort to your existing behaviors such as increasing the walking time from 10 minutes to 15 minutes.

Let's compare this approach with someone making a New Year's Resolution to "Lose 30 pounds, cut out all junk food, eat a salad everyday, juice every morning, and exercise 5 times a week in the gym."

If this person doesn't do *any* of those things already, they are going to feel completely overwhelmed. They may get a good start with their initial burst of motivation, but eventually work, family, friends, and other priorities get in the way and there's about a 95%+ chance they're going to give up.

Now compare this to someone who simply decides that for their first month, they're going to cut out their afternoon snack and replace it with a piece of fruit.

The second month they're going to exercise *at least* twice a week for 20 minutes, starting with home workouts in front of the TV so they can still catch their favorite shows.

The third month they add in a salad for lunch and now go to the gym at least twice a week. So on and so fourth.

By the end of the year, they could easily have lost 30 pounds, dramatically reduced their junk food intake, and most importantly have made *long-standing* changes to their habits. Their new behaviors were gradually introduced into their life so they weren't overwhelmed. They chose actions that were challenging, but still manageable enough that they knew they could stick with them long enough for them to become habitual.

Not only has the second person achieved their goals, but as I've seen in my experience, they'll likely continue these behaviors year after year and actually get to keep their results.

Remember, what comes quickly can be lost quickly. What comes from persistence remains *persistently.*

2: The Best Trick To Overcome Any Excuse

Henry Ford says "whether you believe you can or can't, you're right." One of the biggest roadblocks to fitness success that I've seen in both myself and others are the limiting beliefs someone can tell themselves like "I don't have enough time" "I don't have enough money" "I can't stop myself from eating junk food" "I hate exercise" etc.

When a person tells themselves these things, their brain will literally not let them see any other alternative. And I've found it doesn't really do someone any good to tell some "just think positively" without showing them how to actually go inside their brain and change their beliefs.

The technique I'm going to share with you is my #1 technique to overcome excuses, unlock creative problem solving abilities, and will ideally be used in every area of your life you want to improve. If you took this piece of advice and ran with it, I believe it could be *the* answer to everything that you feel is holding you back. That's not an exaggeration. This technique is what changed many areas of my life, not just my health.

Before I understood how the brain worked, I would often tell myself things like "I hate healthy food and I can't give up my favorite fast food meals." Then I realized that these sorts of beliefs are created and reinforced by the language that runs through the mind, often subconsciously.

Each day we tell and ask ourselves all sorts of things. These things could be "I don't have enough time." "I'm a failure." "Why can't I overcome my junk food cravings?"

Or alternatively...

"I can make time to exercise twice this week" "I am successful" "What do I love about eating healthy foods?"

The one thing I've found can turn everything around is simply changing one's language patterns from dis-empowering statements and dis-empowering questions to instead asking high quality *questions.*

One reason this technique works is because *I* can't tell *you* what will work best for *your* life. Instead, the best answers and solutions for you will always come from within yourself, even if it takes the help of someone else to draw it out of you.

Here's an experiment. Try saying these things to yourself and see how you feel:

- "I don't know what to do."
- "Everything is hopeless."
- "Why is there never enough time?"
- "What is wrong with me?

Be honest with yourself, even if you haven't ever made these exact statements in your own life, have you ever told or asked yourself something that made things seem impossible or extremely difficult? Have these things ever at times been things that you really knew weren't totally true?

Let's replace these with with "empowering questions." See how you feel when asking these things:

- "What's one simple thing that I **can** do right now to start moving me forward even more?"
- "What can I do with the time I do have?"
- "What healthier foods *do* I enjoy?"
- "How can I make healthier foods taste even better?"
- "Why am I getting even more fit each day?"
- "How can I make getting fit even more enjoyable?"
- "How can I do the best that I can?"

Now, as a tip, try asking questions that can improve your outlook on life in general like:

- "When have I been successful in the past?"
- "How does it get even better than this?"

- "Why is everything working out for the best even if I can't see it?"

Let's take the sample question: "What's one simple thing that I **can** do right now to start moving me forward even more?"

The answer doesn't have to be something big. Maybe it's just doing 5 jumping jacks in the morning or replacing a candy bar with a piece of fruit.

Then keep asking the question regularly and build up more and more. One could then ask "could I do 10 jumping jacks a day **and** add in 10 pushups?" If the answer is yes, one would do that.

When that is comfortable, one would ask themselves "could I go *even further?*"

Not all questions will have an obvious answer right away. Let's say you ask "how can I make exercise extremely fun?" and you don't come up with an answer. Some questions will either not have a clear answer, or will be too outside of your current knowledge zone for you to determine a solution.

Then try another question like "how can I make exercise *at least a little more* enjoyable?"

Perhaps that's by listening to an audio book while exercising or setting up a friendly competition with others with prizes for whoever makes the most progress in their exercise routine. The great thing is, whatever answer you come up with will be *your own*.

The point of this is not that asking one question will solve all your problems just like one workout won't get you a dream body. It's the <u>consistent</u> practice and making it a habit that *will* change your life.

Thomas Edison failed over 1000 times when creating the light bulb. The reason he succeeded is because inventors are naturally curious.

He said that each failure was a *success* in getting closer to finding a solution. Rather than saying "I messed up, I'm a failure." Or asking "why do I never succeed?" He may have asked "given

17

that this didn't work, what can I do differently that will move me closer to creating this light bulb?" "What do I need to learn or try to make this work?" Etc.

What you focus on expands!

If that's problems, you'll see more problems. If that's potential *solutions* to problems, you'll start to see more *solutions*. Not always right away, but eventually the brain will start to see new things and make connections that you could have never thought of before.

Here's another example:

"What's one healthier food I can enjoy, afford, and have time to eat?"

Perhaps that's just eating one apple a day. If that's all you can do to change your diet for the next month, that's great! Even if one still eats a bunch of junk food, the point is not to get the perfect diet over night. It's to be in the practice of **constant** forward motion and growth so that, a year later, one has made a noticeable difference. (It will likely happen much sooner though!)

No matter how seemingly insignificant the step forward is, it will start to snowball. This is more about changing psychology and language patterns than it is one's physical body at first. Apply this to every area of your life, and it will be impossible for it not to change for the better.

Use your own questions and you'll discover your own answers.

This advice is worth more than gold if you truly apply it to your life.

If struggling to find a good question, you can always ask yourself "what's a good question to ask?"

In all my years of studying health, psychology, and personal development, I've found this simple insight: **The answer is a question.**

3: How To Stay Motivated

I'm going to let you in on a big secret to motivation...

You don't need to *get* motivated - you're *already* motivated.

It's just that sometimes we can be *more* motivated to eat desserts than vegetables or watch a TV show than exercise.

The issue isn't *getting* motivated, it's figuring out how to **redirect** where our motivation lies.

What motivates us are three basic things. Pain, pleasure, and love. While having an unhealthy body can cause physical pain and being in great shape can cause physical pleasure, for the most part with health and fitness, it's more about psychological pain and pleasure.

Everything you do, healthy or not, stems from the fact that psychologically it is meeting one of your six human needs. Those needs are certainty/security, variety/excitement, love/connection, significance/control, growth, and contribution. Meet these needs and feel pleasure. Don't meet them and feel pain.

The reason why it's hard for people to give up their favorite foods and old habits is because those habits meet one or more of those six human needs. That means if you want to get *more* motivated to do something else like eat healthier and exercise, you'll need to mentally connect the dots of how those new behaviors (and the outcomes like a more fit body) will <u>also</u> satisfy those emotional needs to an equal or greater extent.

I cover this in depth in my book How To Stick To A Diet (excuseproof.com/diet) where I go over four human needs (leaving out contribution and growth as they're not as heavily diet related). But you don't need an in-depth understanding of your psychology to know how to redirect your motivation. You already do this whether you're conscious of it or not. But if you want to have conscious control over it, here's an exercise.

1. Write down all the short term and long term problems (pains) with continuing to engage in an undesired behavior. (Eating junk food, not exercising, etc.)

Examples of these problems could be lacking energy, disease and sickness, weight gain, etc. It's also critical to ask why *those* things would be a problem. This could mean not being there for one's family, not being able to pursue a passion, feeling out of control of one's life, etc.

2. Write down all the short term and long term benefits (pleasures) with engaging in a desired behavior. (Eating healthier, exercising, etc.)

Examples of these benefits could be more energy, a sexy body, less aches and pains, not having to take prescription drugs, etc.

It's also critical to ask **why** you want those things until you tap into how they meet your needs for more certainty, variety, connection, significance, contribution, and/or growth.

For instance, a person that is very family oriented may connect eating healthier with being a better spouse and parent by improving their health, living longer, and setting a good example. This would meet their connection, certainty, and contribution needs.

It's important to keep asking "why?" for every reason you can come up with for wanting your goals until you hit upon a reason that truly moves you and fills you with passion.

For instance, if someone is considering why they want to eat better, they may say: "To be healthier" "Why do I want to be healthier?" "So I don't die an early death." "Why am I worried about an early death?" "Because if I don't eat healthier, my doctor says I'm on a fast track to heart disease and that means I won't get to see my kids graduate and get married. I can't stand the thought of not being there for my family."

People who make great changes to their body and their lives don't do so because they just "kind of felt like it." They make great changes because they reached a tipping point where they realized it was too painful, or *would be* too painful to remain the same.

They had a huge reason why, and you must keep asking yourself why you want to be more healthy and fit until you come up with reasons that inspire a *burning passion* to take control of your habits.

Doing this exercise is powerful in itself, but I've found a way that helps me remember my motivations day in and day out when any temptations pop up.

That is by asking myself an empowering question in the form of "would I rather..."

Let's say I see some ice cream (my favorite snack) at the store and am tempted to buy it. I would simply ask myself "would I rather eat this ice cream and feel like crap by depressing my immune system with massive amounts of sugar and adding fat to my body **OR** would I rather buy some fruit to satisfy my sweet tooth and feel good about myself knowing that I am giving my body the nutrients it needs while maintaining a lean physique?"

4: The #1 Cause Of Fitness Failure

What either causes or aggravates almost every single disease?

I'll give you a hint, it's not a poor diet, lack of exercise, or having "bad" genetics.

When I discovered the true impact of this one thing, I was blown away because I realized that most health and fitness experts rarely mention how to address it despite the fact that it is the *biggest* factor on a person's health and fitness and almost everyone suffers from its effects. To make matters worse, failure to take care of this one thing will also lead to reduced willpower, a depressed immune system, and a general lack of happiness even if one <u>does</u> reach their fitness goals.

So I've made it my mission to spread awareness about this.

That one thing is *excess* stress (or prolonged negative emotions). While a little bit of stress is beneficial (think exercise), too much stress creates a series of conditions in the body that lead to disease, aging, and even gaining stubborn belly fat due to excess cortisol. It saps the body of energy, and it leads to feelings of being overwhelmed.

The thing is, every new action a person takes on will create a bit of a stress response. Under healthy conditions, this is easily managed and beneficial. But when a person is stressed out with work, family, and other commitments, something as simple as changing one's lunch or starting an exercise routine can be all it takes for the body to say "no more!"

If you've ever had times in your life where you welcomed challenges and felt like you can take on the world, this is the natural willpower and strength that resides in you when it's not being sapped dealing with too many daily stressors. If you don't feel like you have that kind of willpower right now, don't worry. It's not necessarily because you're inherently weak willed. It's more likely because you're either physically, emotionally, or psychologically stressed out.

Many of the tips in this guide will help make the process of staying healthy and fit less stressful, but what about the current stress that's in your life?

There are four big things that have dramatically reduced stress in my life. The next three tips on sleep, meditation, and mindfulness are critical for stress management, but this tip I'm about to share with you is quite possibly the easiest and yet most overlooked way of reducing stress.

Before I learned this, I oftentimes used to find myself feeling overwhelmed with all of the things I needed to do. It was like my brain was overflowing with racing thoughts trying to hold onto everything until I reached points where I would simply sit back, watch TV, and do *nothing* because as soon as I thought about the things I had to do, I would be so overwhelmed it was paralyzing.

That is until I threw out my to-do list, and made a priority list. The method of prioritization I use is simple.

1. Write down everything you want and need to do. Simply getting it on paper reduces the mental clutter because it allows you to not have to worry about forgetting anything.

2. Write down what is most important for the short term I.E. Your short term goals. This obviously should include your physical fitness and health goals.

3. Write down weekly and daily action steps that must be done to reach those goals. For myself, this is typically only 2-4 things per day on a dry-erase board I keep on my desk in constant sight. Everything I have to do during the day is secondary to those things. For example: "Exercise for 30 minutes" "Cook a vegetable stew"

I suggest taking care of these things, when at all possible, before anything else that is secondary.

For some, this could mean exercising first thing in the morning before other distractions could get in the way. And when a priority doesn't get done on a day, it is rescheduled if at all possible or additional effort is made later in the week to compensate. This isn't always possible, but a good thing to strive for.

The big thing with stress reduction is when going about my day and my mind would start to race with thoughts of things that *were* priorities, but not priorities *right now*, I would make a note (on phone, through simpleology.com or evernote.com, or paper) to take care of it later.

Remember that while you can't handle *everything*, you can handle *anything* **one thing at a time**.

5: Secrets To Serene Sleep

Sleep deprivation is a form of torture that is effective at not only making a person miserable, but it was used heavily on prisoners of war because it's very good at doing another thing – reducing willpower.

So do you think if a person lacks sleep and therefore willpower they might be more prone to give into junk food cravings?

The answer of course is YES! But that's only scratching the surface. Let's look at many of the reasons why sleep is kind of a big deal.

Lack of sleep can cause junk food binging.

healthland.time.com/2012/06/11/why-sleepy-people-reach-for-junk-food

Lack of sleep slows metabolism and increases cortisol which can lead to weight gain.

www.sciencedaily.com/releases/1999/10/991025075844.htm

Lack of sleep depresses the immune system making sickness more likely.

http://articles.mercola.com/sites/articles/archive/2012/06/02/can-sleeping-affect-immune-system.aspx

Lack of sleep is associated with increases in depression.

http://healthland.time.com/2010/09/02/lack-of-sleep-can-cause-depression-weight-gain-and-even-death/

Sleep is necessary to grow brain cells and establish new learning.

www.livescience.com/16966-sleep-brain-learn-nsf-ria.html

I point a few of the many reasons why sleep is critical because some people feel like sleep is the one thing they can afford to sacrifice, and yet it may be one of the most fundamental things for a healthy body, healthy relationships, and an overall happy life. Probably not things you want to give up, right?

For anyone who *doesn't* want to be overweight, sick, depressed, weak, dumbed down, more prone to accidents and injuries, miserable, and die at a younger age, here are some tips you can do to maximize your sleep and enjoy a happy and fit body:

The first and most critical thing to mention is to sleep grounded. I thought about making an entire section on the health benefits of grounding (earthing) alone. What grounding does is allows you to absorb negatively charged free electrons. These electrons act as antioxidants, reduce inflammation, and will normalize circadian rhythms effectively balancing cortisol levels. Grounding is also associated with significant pain reduction. The body is electrical as well as chemical, and it's been speculated all the electronic devices in modern times can throw off the body's electrical systems. Grounding prevents electromagnetic radiation (which comes from computers, cell phones, and other electronic devices) from negatively affecting the body. It is quite possibly the "missing link" to good health.

See the book "Earthing" by Clinton Ober and Steven Sinatra at www.amazon.com/Earthing-Most-Important-Health-Discovery/dp/1591202833 and also visit EarthingInstitute.net to read about this incredible discovery. Inexpensive grounding mats or bed sheets may be purchased to sleep on at Earthing.com/Shop_s/1824.htm. I suggest simply purchasing the "Universal Mat," and using it both during the day and sleeping on it at bedtime which is what I do.

Magnesium deficiency is extremely common and leads to insomnia. I suggest using magnesium oil or 500 mg of chelated magnesium daily as well as foods rich in magnesium like nuts and seeds.

Reduce exposure to artificial light and stimulating things like computers and TVs before bed as light exposure can interfere with the production of melatonin. Melatonin is needed for proper sleep and relaxation. You can run a free program on your computer called F.lux which will effectively dim computer screens to match the background environment and helps prevent the screen from keeping you awake. Get it at stereopsis.com/flux. Inexpensive glasses can be worn for nighttime TV watching that block out blue spectrum light so you can still watch TV without disrupting melatonin production. Get them at www.amazon.com/Uvex-S1933X-Eyewear-SCT-Orange-Anti-Fog/dp/B000USRG90. Dim bedroom lights if possible. Wear a sleeping mask if needed. Make sure windows are covered to prevent excess sun exposure or light exposure if an issue in the mornings. Reading or meditation is a good way to wind down. Foam ear plugs help if there's a lot of noise.

Valerian, Passion Flower, and Chamomile help to calm the nerves and relax. Passion flower in particular is a great herb to calm the nerves that many people aren't aware of, but it is highly recommended for anxiety. Try making one of these as an herbal tea or take a quality extract. 5-htp, l-theanine, and melatonin or a high quality supplement like "Sleep Wizard" (www.drdavesbest.com/products/sleep-wizard.html) may also help.

6: How To Grow Your Brain And Change Your Genes

What if there is actually a way to grow your brain, alter your genetics, and make stress a thing of the past?

Neuroscientists in recent years have discovered something called neuroplasticity which basically says the brain can change its structure and grow various regions of the brain in response to stimulus. But like a muscle, the brain is a "use it or lose it" sort of organ. The benefit for fitness is that the brain can be trained to make the body more resilient to stress and therefore potentially improve health and appearance.

With regards to genetics, we've also discovered in recent years the phenomena of epigenetics. While you can't change your actual genetic code, environmental factors like diet, toxic exposure, and all the various stressors can determine which genes "turn on and off" so to speak. That means you're **not** doomed to get a disease or suffer an ailment just because it runs in your family.

Learn about epigenetics here: excuseproof.com/epigenetics

What's most exciting is that research shows not only how we can prevent aging and disease, but actually turn on genes associated with good health to counteract the damaging effects of one's environment. This tip and the following are designed to create a beneficial change in your epigenetics.

The first technique is good old mindfulness meditation which now has numerous scientific studies showing the benefits for reducing stress as well as altering the brain, genes, and behavior.

The simplest meditation is a breathing mindfulness meditation where you:

- Sit in a relaxed upright position with your spine straight and feet flat on the floor. Alternatively, if you're comfortable in a seated meditation position you may do that.
- Start to focus on your breathing in and out. No need to change your breathing, just observe it.

- If it helps you relax, you can mentally "scan" your body head to toe relaxing each part.
- Continue this for 1-15 minutes (start with just a few minutes daily), or as long as comfortable.
- As you get more proficient in being able to focus only on your breath during meditation, you may begin to simply observe your thoughts coming and going. Rather than "fighting" any thoughts, simply watch them occur and pass through your awareness. It can help to think of yourself not as "me" or "my thoughts," but as an overall awareness of those things.
- While the purpose of meditation isn't necessarily to try to stop thoughts but rather "observe" them, if you really want to quiet your mind, you may mentally make the effort to "watch for" the next thought that is going to occur. Ironically, the more you try to watch for the next thought to arise, the less thoughts seem to come until your mind becomes quiet and still.

Even though meditation is an active process, don't worry about "screwing it up" and remember as long as you do it regularly, even if your mind wanders a lot at first, you'll start to get better.

Here are some more resources from Zen Habits on how to meditate and make it part of your life:

www.zenhabits.net/meditate

http://zenhabits.net/meditation-for-beginners-20-practical-tips-for-quieting-the-mind

www.zenhabits.net/build-strength

As a bonus, for those interested in growing parts of the brain associated with developing a higher IQ and other mental benefits, check out this article and free software:

www.bulletproofexec.com/how-to-add-2-75-iq-points-per-hour-of-training

brainworkshop.sourceforge.net

7: Become Happier To Become Healthier

There is a part of your body that may be even more important with regards to your mood and emotions than your brain.

Researchers have found this organ actually sends signals to the brain which the brain responds to. When this organ doesn't function optimally due to stress, it sends a signal to the brain that can depress the immune function for several hours. But with a simple technique researchers have discovered, this organ can send a positive signal to the brain that triggers healing and vitality. Many people have reported improvements in chronic health conditions by applying this one simple technique.

That organ is the heart and the research being done on it comes from the Heartmath Institute at Heartmath.org. They've been able to measure something called Heart Rate Variability and make associations between HRV and various health conditions in the body. The simplest explanation is that a high HRV (which is termed coherence) is created when one is in a low to no stress state and feeling positive emotions such as love, joy, gratitude, care, forgiveness, etc.

On the contrary, when there's a low HRV (which many people in modern stressful times experience chronically), the immune system gets depressed and the body breaks down. In essence, your emotions (tied to stress) play as much or more of a role in your health than your diet and exercise do!

What's even more amazing is that the heart emits a measurable electromagnetic field. We can subconsciously pick up on a person's heart rate pattern when we're in their presence. Researchers have been able to prove this and provide a scientific explanation as to why you can get good or bad "vibes" from someone whenever they walk into a room. The age old idea of your heart being where your emotions reside and the value of listening to your heart has gathered a lot of scientific confirmation.

Here's a simple exercise to reduce stress and create a high HRV state. This can be done in combination with a meditation practice or on its own.

- Place your hand on your heart and imagine your breathe coming in and out of the heart area.
- Bring your focus to the present moment. Imagine your heart pulling in all scattered thoughts and feelings.
- Think of anything that brings feelings of joy, care, and/or gratitude. I myself focus on gratitude and ask "What am I grateful for?""Why am I grateful for these things?""What should I be grateful for?"
- Allow yourself to simply relax into the feeling of your heart and these positive emotions for 5-10 minutes as best as you can. It's ok if it doesn't come naturally at first. With regular practice this will become easier. You're training yourself to enter into a higher HRV state more readily and more often without any effort.

For more stress reduction tips and strategies, I suggest checking out the free de-stress kit from Heartmath at heartmath.com/destresskit.

Also check out the book "The Heartmath Solution" which can be purchased at excuseproof.com/resources/recommended-books.

For more tips on gratitude, check out my youtube video at excuseproof.com/gratitude

Here is a great article for those who find traditional gratitude practices ineffective and how to get more use out of them: ArtOfManliness.com/2012/12/03/the-george-bailey-technique

8: Health Success Hides Here

If you fell down a hole, knocked yourself out, and woke up to find yourself surrounded by total darkness not remembering how you got there, what would be the first thing you need to know to escape?

It would be the *awareness* that you're in a hole.

Awareness is the first step in making a change.

And yes, you should want to know how to make a change in your life. I want to point this out because some people think "I don't need to change. I like myself as I am and don't want to be someone else."

As critical as it is to accept yourself as you are, it's also important to recognize that nothing in nature stays the same. An oak tree will never become an apple tree just like you will never become someone you're not, but that oak will also never be the *exact same* oak tree from one year to the next. It will be growing or dying, have more or less leaves, etc.

So the question is, if you're going to change from one day to the next regardless of whether or not you want to, do you want to leave the change that happens to you in your life up to chance or choice?

The reason why we tend to get "stuck" (and seemingly *not* change) however is we can get caught in various "holes" of bad habits, dis-empowering thoughts, and limiting beliefs without even being *aware* of it.

Without **practicing** awareness (which can also be called mindfulness, presence, or living in the "now"), a person is simply like a robot running on autopilot following programmed routines and habits without much conscious thought.

A more everyday example of this would be driving in a car, and then not remembering the last few minutes of driving only to "snap back to reality" and realize that somehow or another, you've safely driven the past few miles without even being aware of it.

Or perhaps eating an entire tub of ice cream and then looking back and going, "Wow! How did that happen?"

All of these instances, from the more deep trances of driving and TV watching, to the more everyday decisions of what to eat result from the habitual way our brain works. Over 90% of our decisions are made without any conscious effort or deep understanding *why* we made those decisions in the moment. In essence, the feeling that you are always aware of your thoughts and rationalizations for making most of your decisions is an **illusion**.

Awareness is quite simply observing your thoughts and feelings without judgment. Nothing is labeled as right or wrong, it's just "interesting." You become both a participant and observer of your life. This practice is powerful because it teaches you that you are not your thoughts and feelings. You are simply that which is *aware* of thoughts and feelings that flow *through you*. I remind myself of this by asking "am I this thought or feeling, or am I simply that which is *aware* of it?"

Awareness / mindfulness requires being present. This is critical because the only point in time where a person can change anything is *now*. Your past can be reinterpreted *right now*. Your present can change with any choice you make *right now*. And your future is determined by what you do *right now*.

In other words, success and opportunity hide in the very place people are sometimes distracting themselves from - **the present moment**.

Opportunity is here with you in this very moment as soon as you choose to let go of thinking about the past and future and notice what is here with you in this moment.

To practice awareness or mindfulness, simply notice all your thoughts and feelings as they occur throughout the day without judging them. You may be surprised at what you learn and how you start to change without even trying.

By actually practicing awareness, you can start to notice your habitual thoughts, feelings, and underlying beliefs behind every action you take. The biggest trick with awareness is that you're not actually trying to change your behaviors, thoughts, or feelings when you're observing them. A person may go ahead and eat an entire tub of ice cream, but they should notice all of their thoughts, feelings, and everything they are experiencing before, during, and after eating the ice cream.

While this may sound odd at first, consider that this person eating the ice cream may discover how they didn't want to eat the ice cream because they were physically hungry, but rather because they're experiencing an emotional emptiness inside. The ice cream was satisfying an emotional want, not a physical one. Being aware of this is the first step to breaking the pattern, and sometimes it takes nothing more than awareness to break the pattern.

But awareness isn't just a one time thing, it should be an on-going practice. One of the benefits of practicing meditation is that is helps the brain become trained to me more present and mindful at all times. In a sense, awareness is taking meditation to your everyday life so everything you do becomes meditation. This has been promoted for thousands of years as a spiritual practice for one big reason – it works.

9: Making Mistakes For More Motivation

One of the biggest stumbling blocks I see people make is letting a few mistakes completely take them out of the game. They'll make statements like: "I messed up my diet this meal, so today is ruined. I'll just get back on track tomorrow." Or "I didn't make it to the gym for the last three days so I'll start over again next week."

When I hear this stuff, to me it's the equivalent of someone saying "I wasn't able to take a shower today so I might as well not even bother showering for the rest of the week." If health and fitness is a habit/lifestyle (as I encourage people to make it), mistakes are to be *expected* as both part of the process of learning and as part of being human.

I'm going to share with you my simple process for not only overcoming the fear of making mistakes, but to actually welcome them and use them as a way to get even **more** motivated and excited.

The first step is simple acceptance that you *will* make mistakes. The second step is to re-frame mistakes as potential *successes* in learning. A lot of the world's most successful people, whether in fitness, business, or other areas, were successful because they A) made mistakes and B) learned lessons from those mistakes they could have never otherwise learned had they not been willing to fail.

Tell yourself right now "I'm going to screw things up, and that's ok! A mistake isn't the end, it's just an opportunity to learn how to do better going forward."

When a mistake is made, some empowering questions to ask are: "What can I learn from this?" "How can I prevent this from happening again?" "Why is everything still ok?"

Your success is not determined by how many times you fall

35

down, but by how quickly you get back up. And the more times you fall, the more "practice" you can have at getting up quicker each time.

Another way to handle mistakes is to realize it's not about the end goal as much as it is the process of *striving for* your goals that really matters. "It's about the journey and not the destination" or "it's a marathon, not a sprint" are statements that have unfortunately become cliche, but they express a profound truth.

Another quote that really sums it up for me comes from Zig Ziglar who says "what you get by reaching your goals is not nearly as important as what you *become* by reaching them."

Some people are so obsessed about reaching their goal that seems so far away they feel like they can't be happy until they're there. But I'll let you in on a secret, there is no "there." There only is and ever will be **now**. You can only be learn, be happy, or experience anything else in this present moment.

If you can embrace and focus on what you enjoy about the process (which will include both mistakes and successes) of growing and developing into your fullest potential, you'll find you can be happy and motivated each and every day *regardless* of your body's current condition.

10: What Force Is Stronger Than Willpower?

There seems to be one thing I've found consistently that separates those who are successful in sticking to their resolutions and those who give up.

See if you can figure out for yourself why "Jim" is successful at reaching his fitness goals and "Bob" eventually gives up.

Bob is serious about making a change. He writes down his goals and has set up a diet plan based on tips he remembers hearing years ago. The first step is he will bring in a salad every day to lunch. His co-workers, who don't share his same enthusiasm for good health, joke around with Bob about how Bob is has turned into a "health nut." Bob also is serious about working out and has gotten himself a nice home gym setup. He has an old book he picked up on doing home bodyweight workouts and he is determined to follow through. Which he does... for a while.

Jim is equally serious. He invests some money in getting an online fitness coach. The coach provides a good body weight workout routine Jim can do at home (very similar to Bob's). They talk about his goals, and he writes an action plan for success that they go over. Jim also brings in a salad to work, but he eats it by himself so he can focus on listening to an audio book on nutrition. Each week Jim checks in with his coach on his progress.

Both Bob and Jim have set similar goals, follow a similar workout routine, made similar changes to their diets, and both have access to quality information on how to get fit.

But Bob fails while Jim succeeds. Why is this?

I'll give you a hint, it's the same reason why someone in the military will push themselves beyond their usual limits. It's the same reason a stay at home mom will make incredible sacrifices for her children. It's the same reason why a person will work tirelessly at a job they don't enjoy when they have bills to pay.

The difference is the environment.

Yogananda expresses this with the simple statement that "environment is stronger than willpower."

We are influenced to a strong degree by our environment. This is because we have something built into our biology called called "mirror neurons." Mirror neurons literally recreate, in our minds, what we experience externally with our senses. These mirror neurons may be why seeing someone yawn can make you yawn. Or hearing others laugh can make you want to laugh.

What this means for sticking with a fitness habit, or any other habit for that matter, is that your environment and things like accountability may have more to do with success than your willpower.

You see, Bob was facing two issues. The first is that he wasn't accountable to anyone like a coach or partner who he could check in with to keep him on track. He worked out at home which is fine, but he didn't have anyone to push him or make sure he followed through with his workouts. He also didn't invest much time or money into his success so he didn't feel bad when he gave up.

His environment at work was also an issue. He was eating lunch with people who constantly teased him about getting healthy rather than supporting his decision. He really was going in it alone.

Jim on the other hand hired a coach. This meant he had to invest time and money in his success so he was sure to make it worth his sacrifice. This also meant he had someone who he checked in with that was making sure he was following through with his home workout routines and providing inspiration.

Jim put himself into a positive environment at work too. Jim knew his co-workers, like Bob's, wouldn't understand why he's decided to eat healthier. So he simply decides to take that time to separate himself from potential negative influences and instead put himself in a positive environment of learning more about health by listening to an audio book.

Let's look at a few examples of a poor environment for fitness success:

- Having a kitchen stocked full of foods that you wish to avoid.

- Eating out at places that will put tempting foods in front of you.

- Exercising with people who don't push themselves at all.

- Sharing your goals and accomplishments with people who will criticize you or not support you.

- Hanging out with others who don't share similar goals and ambitions.

None of these things are *inherently* bad.

It would be impossible to always avoid tempting foods. It would also be particularly difficult to always avoid people who won't support you, especially when they are family, co-workers, and close friends.

But the idea here is that you'll want to be aware of these things having an influence, and either minimize your exposure to them, and/or compensate with more positive influences in your environment.

There are many ways to set up your environment for success, here are a few:

- Hanging out with peers whom you aspire to be like. Visit Meetup.com to find local meetup groups related to health, fitness, and physical activities you enjoy. This helps creates both accountability and makes the process of staying fit more enjoyable when you share the experience with others.

- Having a mentor or a coach who both teaches and keeps you accountable.

- Having the right kinds of foods in your kitchen.
- Visual cues like inspirational pictures and quotes.

- Reading books and stories about people you admire.
- Reading, listening to, or watching educational material.
- Engaging in visualization to see and feel your goals as a reality.

The take home point here is that if you have limited willpower, that willpower is best invested in setting up a positive environment rather than wasted on having to fight against a poor environment.

It's very important to have positive influences for belief building too. Many barriers are mental, and oftentimes it takes seeing someone else break through a barrier before we believe we can do it ourselves. This is why a mentor is so helpful, but even hearing inspiring true stories can help.

It's also important to note that just because one has environmental influences that are "negative" doesn't mean they're doomed to fail. Going back to empowering questions, one can ask themselves "how can I make my environment a little better?" "Why will I succeed no matter what obstacles I face?"

The most powerful solution I've ever found whenever I catch myself letting other people's opinions or criticism bring me down is asking this simple question: "Do I want to let other people's opinions have power over me, or would I keep my power to reach my goals and live on my own terms?"

11: How To Handle Unwanted Emotions

Even the most rational human beings are basically driven by emotions. That means your actions stem from your emotions and are usually only later justified by logic.

So what does someone do if their emotions aren't doing them any favors? What if someone's emotions drive them to binge eating? Or playing video games for the 7th hour straight instead of exercising? Or feeling depressed about the way their body looks and feels?

Aren't emotions something that happen to us beyond our control?

There are a handful of tips in this book that I consider "life changing." These are the tips that, even if I didn't truly fathom their significance at first, once I applied them <u>regularly</u> in my life, I was never the same after.

The tip I'm about to share with you is the blueprint (we should have been taught in school) on how to handle emotions and the ability to simply "let go" of any emotions.

"Letting go" is a very simple but life changing process. It is essentially the ability we all have to let go of or "release" any feelings, beliefs, attachments, resistances that we have internally. Mastering this technique can give you <u>complete emotional freedom</u>.

Here are some examples of "letting go." A little kid has a fight with his friend, and five minutes later they're playing together like nothing happened. An adult gets cut off in traffic, and five minutes later they've forgotten about it and are chatting with a friend.

But, if these people didn't "let it go," the person who got cut off ends up chasing the other driver down the highway with a bad case of road rage. Or that kid grows up and still broods over that one time Timmy called him a "stupid face."

Sometimes people confuse "letting go" with suppressing

emotions or "pretending" like nothing is wrong when "letting go" is quite the opposite. You instead **welcome** your thoughts and feelings without trying to fight them.

So if you feel like crying – cry. I would suggest doing this exercise alone at first. As you get better, you can let go on the spot such as in a heated environment. In fact, letting go is powerful for keeping your cool and thinking clearly in high stress situations.

One very simple process of letting go is:

1. Welcome and accept all thoughts and feelings without judgment or resistance.
2. Ask yourself, "can I let this go?" "would I let this go?" "would I rather hold onto this or be free?"
3. Repeat the process of welcoming the thoughts and feelings and asking if you could let it go.

Why does this work?

Because instead of fighting against the emotions, you're welcoming them. Emotions are like someone knocking on the door who will keep knocking until you welcome them in, let them have their say, and then they tend to just leave all on their own.

Another aspect of letting go is forgiveness. Now just to be clear, forgiveness **is** a health and fitness topic because the research clearly shows that holding onto anger, resentment, and negative emotions from the past eats away at the body.

There's a quote on forgiveness, which to paraphrase, says "holding resentment is like drinking poison and waiting for the other person to die."

Holding onto anger, resentment, and not forgiving is taking your body, health, and happiness prisoner. You'll never be free to truly live as you want and experience the fullness of life. And to be clear, forgiveness includes forgiving yourself.

I and no one else but yourself can make you forgive. It's beyond the scope of this guide to touch on how to forgive those who've done serious wrong. To forgive what some people have done can quite literally be the hardest thing a person can do, but at the same time the most rewarding in its ability to lift a heavy emotional burden.

I simply ask myself, "would I rather hold onto this and feel pain, or would I rather just let it go and be free? Is this really worth losing my inner peace over, or would I rather just let it go?" "Why am I able to forgive this person?" "Why am I able to forgive even more now?"

It might not happen right away, but slowly but surely with enough of going through this process each day, I can let go of resentment, let go of judgment, and simply be at peace with what is as no amount of wishing things to be different will make it so.

For self forgiveness, if possible, reach out to others and sincerely apologize. It's not important about whether they forgive you, but recognizing your own mistakes, owning up to them, and forgiving yourself. This can also mean telling yourself you're sorry for how you've treated yourself or your body.

This may sound very "spiritual" for a fitness book, but there is no separating this stuff from the health of the body. I could talk about diet tips and exercise tips all day long, but if I don't mention this stuff, I'm leaving out something that has a far greater impact on your health and happiness than getting a six pack.

For more information on "letting go" and emotional management, I highly recommend you read the book "The Sedona Method" by Hale Dwoskin which is the best resource I've found on the topic. This book alone will likely give you all you need to successfully stick to your fitness goals from an "emotional" point of view in addition to resolving many other emotional issues and addictions a person may have.

The bestselling book "The Power Of Now" by Eckhart Tolle is another excellent read for understanding acceptance and non-resistance on a deeper level from a more philosophical/spiritual view. See: excuseproof.com/resources/recommended-books

If you have any long standing emotional trauma, it's worth everything to seek counseling and help in order to let those things go and find forgiveness.

12: How To Overcome Emotional Food Cravings

Researchers have sound a simple way to "hack" the brain to cut down on junk food cravings, and all it takes is changing a single word you use.

An LA Times article mentioned simply changing the phrase "I can't" (restrictive) to "I don't" (choice) improves dietary compliance and cuts cravings. See: excuseproof.com/cravings

A reason for this is probably because we as human beings naturally sometimes rebel against anything that will limit our freedom (called reactance in psychology).

But is there a way to make this language shift even more powerful?

I've found for myself there is. That's by combining an empowering question (which also works to override the reactance response) phrased as "would I rather..." and then following it up with the phrase "I choose XYZ because..."

Let's say someone is staring some delicious cookies in the face and they find their willpower wavering. They could ask themselves:

"Would I rather eat these cookies, gain unwanted fat, and not reach my fitness goals OR eat an apple and have a healthy and fit body feeling proud of myself?"

Then follow up with "I choose" and a reason *why* you'll be happier with the healthier choice.

"I choose to eat an apple **because** it will nourish my body, I'll feel great about myself, and I can't wait to see how much more fit I look next week."

If you want to learn more about the psychology behind this and other mind hacks to overcome cravings, check out my book How To Stick To A Diet at excuseproof.com/diet.

13: Inspiration To Change Permanently

Before I did this one thing, I don't think a person could have paid me money to eat a healthy diet. It didn't matter how much my friends and my family were telling me my diet was unhealthy and I needed to change my habits. I was stuck in my ways and nothing seemed to make a difference.

But by doing this one simple thing, I lost just about all of my desire to keep eating that junk food. I *wanted* to eat healthy on my own accord. My desire was so strong that my parents and friends actually thought I was going a little overboard to the other extreme of being *too* health conscious. At that point, a person couldn't pay me to go back to eating junk food and fast food as much as I was.

What I did was expand my awareness through education.

I remember one book that explained how trans-fats and excess sugar affected the body and hormones. This book showed me in black and white terms what was happening to my body internally.

Before that if someone said something was "unhealthy" or "healthy" I didn't really know what that meant. I thought yeah well maybe it's unhealthy because if I keep eating this way for the next 50 years I might get heart disease or something. So I can always change my habits down the road once I had an actual health complication.

Once I had the awareness about the damage I was *currently* doing to my body, I couldn't put on blinders and pretend my habits weren't affecting me.

This of course was just the starting point. There were a number of things that I did that built up my motivation and allowed me to make a more permanent change. But this catalyst really set the pace for everything that came down the road.

I credit part of my ability to stick with a healthy lifestyle for the past nine years straight due to constant on-going education. This is reading articles, books, listening to podcasts, etc. on health and fitness that constantly provide me with reasons why this lifestyle is important, reasons why going back to a less healthy lifestyle are detrimental, and cool tips and tricks that keeps things fun and interesting.

I really believe that when people take even just a few minutes a week to stay up to date on the health impacts of various foods and lifestyle choices, this constant education and reinforcement as to *why* it's important to live healthy is like watering the motivation "plant." If you don't reinforce your motivation by giving it regular "nourishment" (AKA: Reasons "why" health is important), then gradually your motivation starts to die away just like a plant that stops getting watered.

Here are a few health and fitness resources you can check out. There are obviously tons more, but I don't want to overwhelm you. To get started, I suggest signing up for at least one email newsletter and one podcast to keep health education an ongoing weekly thing.

Also, no two experts will always agree with each other, and you may not always agree with them. So I encourage you to take everything with a grain of salt and not get too caught up in "dogmatic" health approaches and simply take and apply what makes sense and works best for you.

Motivational Resources

stronginsideout.com

thechangeblog.com

zenhabits.net

Fitness Resources

excuseproof.com

youtube.com/excuseproof

jcdfitness.com

greatist.com

bodybuilding.com

t-nation.com

Health Resources

mercola.com

renegadehealth.com

thebestdayever.com/news/podcast

bewellbuzz.com and bewellbuzz.com/category/podcast

BulletProofExec.com

Fat, Sick, and Nearly Dead – A documentary on the effects of a poor diet and how they can be reversed through healthier habits like vegetable juicing. Watch for free on Hulu at: http://www.hulu.com/watch/289122

14: Goals – Essential or Overrated?

I'm going to let you in on something that is a little out of the ordinary when it comes to advice on motivation and personal development. Goals are, in many respects, overrated.

Now before anyone gets upset and tells me how important goals are to success, let me give the disclaimer that I love goals and focus heavily on how to properly set and reach goals. I have a goal right now to finish this book by a deadline I've set for myself. I'm also about to give you some little known tricks to significantly increase the likelihood that you'll reach your goals.

The reason why I say goals are "overrated" is not so much because there's anything wrong with goals in themselves, but more something wrong with how some people *view* or *approach* goals. They put goals so high up on a pedestal that they think the goals are the end. They're not.

There is no end, there's only the constant process of growth and development. And if a person isn't growing, they're dying (regressing). Goals are therefore first and foremost a means of prompting one to take on new behaviors and habits or enhance the effectiveness of existing behaviors. Actually *reaching* a goal is **secondary**. Plus, reaching a goal like getting in great shape only to not *stay* in great shape because one hasn't made fitness a lifestyle usually doesn't seem all that appealing to most.

That being said, goals can also be essential at times for gaining clarity and direction for many people, myself included. So in a sense, goals can be *both* essential and overrated depending on the context.

In truth, goals are simply one tool you have for creating change, and some people can do just fine without them while others benefit from them greatly. Some people may be very good at reaching their goals only to not end up being happy when they get there. This is a topic for another book and something I touch on a bit in "How To Stick To A Diet" (excuseproof.com/diet) where I also provide an in-depth explanation of setting and reaching goals.

For now, I'll leave you with these tips on goals:

- Goals are a target to shoot for. It doesn't matter if you don't always hit a bulls eyes, it's more about improving your aim over time.

- Write down your goals on paper. This improves neural connection in the brain. Make sure they're specific and that you know when you've reached them.

- As best as you can, only share your goals with people that will support you and keep you accountable. Research shows that, contrary to popular belief, sharing goals may be detrimental depending on certain factors. There's a power in keeping a secret.

- Make goals present tense by using language like "I am..." instead of "I want to be..." I also like using the phrase "I choose..." which creates a sense of power and confidence.

- Include the positive feelings you'll experience such as happy, excited, grateful, confident, etc.

- Include the habits and behaviors you engage in with your goals rather than just the outcome. EX: "I am so happy I weigh XYZ pounds by choosing to make a vegetable juice for breakfast and exercising 30 minutes 3x a week" vs. simply "I choose to weigh XYZ pounds."

- Use positive rather than negative language in writing your goals. For instance, instead of "I choose to not keep eating junk food," write "I choose to eat healthier foods."

- Use "process" language, especially at first. If "I choose to eat a healthy and nutritious diet" seems unlikely to be accomplished at first, try "I choose to eat even more healthy each day" which makes it more about daily improvements vs. having an ideal diet.

15: Change This, Change Your Life

How is it that I was able to go from eating junk food every night to being a health nut seemingly over night?

While there were things that certainly motivated me to change like learning about the damaging effects of junk food and the benefits of a healthier lifestyle, there are also many people who know that stuff but can't seem to get themselves to make a change. Or at least not a lasting change.

This is part of what lead me on my journey of understanding psychology and neuroscience. On this journey, I discovered an older book that explained it in the simplest terms and made everything click for me.

It explained how the mind works and where our thoughts and behaviors come from on the deepest level. It explained why two people can get surgery to improve the appearance of their bodies, and one will gain confidence while the other would still feel embarassed and ashamed about themselves even if what was "causing" that embarassment originally was removed.

That classic book if you don't already know is called Psycho-Cybernetics by Maxwell Matlz. (excuseproof.com/resources/recommended-books)

The book basically lays out the concept that we act in accord with our self-image. Our self-image is how we perceive ourselves to be. It's our identity we've created in our minds.

The reason why I was able to make a change seemingly overnight is because the first thing I changed was not my behavior, but how I saw myself.

I envisioned my future "ideal" self as being someone that was healthy, fit, and incredibly strong. It was only after I saw this vision and believed it was who I was really capable of being, or more accurately, who I *already* was deep down inside, that my outward actions changed to match that.

One part of a person's self image that often holds them back is they don't believe they are worthy or deserving of what they want.

They beat themselves up with over where they're at.

Although this may make them want to change out of guilt, if a person is in a constant state of self-loathing, it will *not* lead to a lasting nor healthy change.

The first step in changing one's self-image is actually loving acceptance. There's a lot of confusion about what acceptance means. In this case, acceptance doesn't mean accepting your *condition* as being beneficial or impossible to change. It means accepting the simple **reality** of the situation as it is now, and most of all accepting you just as you are now even if you don't plan to stay this way.

In our culture, we often connect a person's worth with their physical appearance, financial status, or external accomplishments such as a job title. This is part of what leads to neurosis and high instances of depression because when one bases their self worth and self image on external things, it's built on a shaky foundation. None of these external things are permanent. Seeking validation, inner peace, and happiness outside of yourself is like trying to find a bus to take you home when you're already at home. The only source of inner peace and happiness exists within you already.

Now some people may think that this acceptance means the same thing as just "staying" with where one is at and not trying to make a change. This is both not the case as well as impossible.

You will change whether you like it or not. All things in nature are either growing or dying. And growth doesn't mean physical growth. Some of the greatest accomplishments and growth a person can experience are when their health is failing and their days are numbered.

In truth, all our days our numbered. So I'll leave you with what I consider to be my most important lesson. Getting healthy and fit is secondary to becoming the best version of yourself that you can be. Having a healthier body allows one to bring their best version of themselves to the world.

The whole point of getting more healthy and fit isn't for striving to be what one's family, friends, or culture says they "ought" to be.

This isn't striving to gain happiness from having a six pack. This isn't striving to live forever.

This is striving to be the best version of *you* that you can be. The version of you that **already** exists within you when you simply recognize it's already there. When you accept that you're perfectly ok just as you are, whereever you are, and that who you are and where you're at will be different tomorrow as you let go of limiting beliefs and fulfill more of your potential.

When you accept that you not only **deserve** to be the best version of you, but the world **needs** it from you.

The only person who can change your life is you. And you already know how to even if you've forgotten.

I'll simply leave you with some questions that may help. But remember, the right question is up to you to find. And the answer is always a question.

- "Can I allow myself to now see the value that I truly have?"
- "Can I allow myself in this moment to simply accept myself as I am right now?"
- "Why do I love and accept myself just as I am now?"
- "What would my ideal self do to be growing even more right now?"
- "Why are all things working for my good?"
- "How can I become an even better version of myself?"
- "What is the lesson here?"
- "What is the lesson I haven't seen until now?"
- "What is the lesson my circumstances are trying to teach me?"
- "Why is everything OK now?"
- "What would my best self do in this situation?"

16: Healthy Meals In A Hurry

One of the biggest obstacles I see people come up against when it comes to eating healthy is a lack of time. If I thought eating better meant spending hours and hours in the kitchen each week cooking and preparing food, I would have given up long ago. And although I'm not as picky as I used to be, if something doesn't taste good, I'm just not going to stick with eating it over the long haul.

It was the challenge of having limited time and a picky taste combined with my desire to eat healthy that led me to a few innovative strategies for eating healthy in a hurry.

The method I'm about to share with you here makes preparing meals from scratch easier, cheaper, tastier, and most of all **faster** than going to fast food places! In fact, I have made healthy meals that lasted for days and took less than 5 minutes to prepare! Sometimes, it would take less than 30 seconds meaning I could, if I wanted to, literally spend less than 1 minute a week preparing meals *from scratch*!

The most effective way I've found for eating healthy on a busy schedule is to use a slow-cooker, also known as a crock-pot. I know the idea of using a slow cooker, which takes 4-8 hours to cook a meal, seems like the exact opposite thing you'd want to use when in a hurry. But bear with me and you'll see why this is exactly what you need.

A slow cooker is great for busy people because it allows you to:

1. Cook in bulk so you can prepare several days worth of food at a time. This means that for an initial 5 minutes of prep time, I often have upwards of 5-10 meals worth of food. This is what makes it faster than fast food as both the original prep-time plus the cleaning and reheating time is super quick.

2. Cook while you're asleep, at work, or just going on about your day by utilizing a slow-cooker with an automatic shut-off.

3. Make just about any kind of great tasting healthy recipe.

My "secret" likes in adjusting slow-cooker recipes to be quicker than usual. I do this by doing a few things:

- I cook food overnight or while at work. My slow cooker has an automatic shut-off so it doesn't matter how long I leave it on for.

- I don't bother to brown meats like some recipes call for. I just toss it in and let it cook.

- Spices and things like onions will have more flavor if added in the last 30 minutes of cooking.

- I occasionally use V8 in place of canned or stewed tomatoes in stews and chili.

- I use a food chopper or mini-blender to save time chopping vegetables. I also use bagged mixed vegetables whenever they're equal in price.

Derek's Quick Crock-pot Chili with Pineapple Recipe:

Ingredients:

- 2lbs of ground or "stew" lean meat (beef, chicken, turkey, bison, etc.)

- 1 can of black beans

- 1 can of kidney beans

- ½ cup of organic brown rice

- 1 cup sliced mushrooms

- 1 cup water

- 3 cups V8 or similar vegetable juice

Spices and Flavors:

- Chili Powder 2 tablespoons – Up to you how much

- 1 tsp of each: Oregano, Basil, Sage, and Thyme. Or just use an Italian seasoning mix.

- Optional: 1 tablespoon minced garlic.

- 20 oz canned pineapples.

Recipe:

1. Add ground lean meat to slow cooker, separate with a fork, and add seasonings. (Don't worry about chopping up too much, you can separate it easier after cooking)

2. Add in ½ cup of dry organic brown rice.

3. Add in 1 cup of water or as much as desired.

4. Open and drain canned beans, add to mix.

5. Add in a cup of pre-sliced mushrooms as well as any other desired vegetables from a bag.

6. Add in various spices and garlic to taste.

7. Mix in up to 3-4 cups of V8 or similar vegetable juice and stir. Alternative: 1 28oz can of diced tomatoes.

8. Cook on high for 3-4 hours or low for 6-8 hours.

9. When finished, taste and add additional spices if desired. You can add 20 oz canned diced pineapples to really kick up the flavor.

Derek's Quick Crock-pot Chicken Curry

Ingredients:

- 1-2 pounds of chicken breast
- 2 cups bagged mixed stir fry vegetables
- 2 cups of rice
- 4 cups of water
- 1 can of unsweetened canned coconut milk (available in ethnic food section)
- 2 tablespoons curry powder
- 1 teaspoon cayenne pepper
- 1 onion
- 1 glove of garlic

Recipe:

1. Add chicken breasts to slow cooker.

2. Add in 2 cups of rice and 4 cups of water.

3. Add in 2 cups of mixed bagged stir fry vegetables.

4. Chop onion then blend with coconut milk, curry powder, garlic, and cayenne pepper to create the curry sauce.

5. Add curry sauce to slow cooker.

6. Cook on high for 3-4 hours or low for 6-8 hours.

See these resources for more information on using a slow cooker:

excuseproof.com/quick-healthy-slow-cooker-chili-recipe-tasty-pineapple-chili

excuseproof.com/healthy-eating-for-busy-people-quick-and-easy-recipes

excuseproof.com/fastchili

17: The Ultimate Salad (For Those Who Hate Salads)

Salads are the stereotypical "health food," and there's good reason for this. Dark leafy greens like spinach, romaine lettuce, and kale are full compounds which enhance health, have cancer fighting benefits, and provide minerals, chlorophyll, and phytonutrients missing in most people's diets.

But there's a problem I faced with greens. No matter how much I knew they were good for me, I hated them and couldn't get myself to eat them on a regular basis. While I could certainly enjoy a nutritionally void iceberg lettuce salad with not so healthy dressings and toppings, I couldn't stomach the truly nutritious salads with dark leafy greens like spinach.

I tried cooking greens, but besides the fact that it takes away some of the health benefits and nutrients (still better than nothing), it still didn't taste that great and I would often end up with a slimy mess.

Then I discovered a way to make raw spinach taste abso-frickin-lutely amazing in only sixty seconds!

I call this "The Sixty Second Salad."

- Take 6-8oz of spinach (can use any leafy green) and put it in a large container.

- Top with a pinch, or about ¼ teaspoon, of unrefined salt.

- Crush the spinach down with hands for about 30 seconds until its condensed.

- Top with a healthy dressing of choice such as any of the following: Salsa, avocado, dried fruit, spices, coconut oil, olives, apple cider vinegar, dijon mustard, etc.

I may also use any healthy homemade sauce which you'll learn about later.

This recipe is great not only because it improves the flavor of the spinach, but also because it condenses it down into a much smaller size making it easy to eat quickly (regular salads take me 10-20 minutes to eat vs. 3-5 for this). The smaller size also makes it extremely portable to stick in a to-go container to take with you on the run.

Add some protein such as canned black beans, tuna, or already cooked meat and you have a complete healthy meal.

Quick, portable, healthy, and most of all tasty! How does it get any better than that?

See me make the 60 second salad here: excuseproof.com/salad

18: You Will Be Addicted To This Healthy Snack

Have you ever eaten salty snacks like potato chips or french fries and found you can't seem to stop yourself from eating them? What if you prepare one of the healthiest foods on the planet in a way that made it just as addicting? If you can do this, then you'll be, in a literal sense, *addicted* to healthy food.

I've found just the way to do that, and that is by making homemade kale chips. Kale chips have started to grow in popularity, but there were a couple of issues I've found with them.

The first is that store bought kale chips are typically super expensive and not ideal for those on a budget.

The second is the homemade kale chip recipes usually call for olive oil and salt. Now olive oil and salt aren't terrible, but I don't like baking with olive oil as it is heat sensitive. I also don't like refined salt as much as an unrefined salt like a Himalayan salt.

So I created kale chips 2.0. These are quicker and easier to make, but feel free to search for any kale chip recipe you enjoy as just getting more kale in your diet is an accomplishment unto itself.

Here's how I make my kale chips which takes about 2 minutes.

- Separate kale from stems or use pre-packaged kale leaves.

- Add curry powder, garlic powder, unrefined salt, and cayenne pepper to taste.

- Bake for 40-50 minutes at 200 degrees or 10-15 minutes at 350 degrees.

See a video here: excuseproof.com/how-to-make-tasty-kale-chips-healthy-snack-recipe & excuseproof.com/kalechips

19: It's Not Just Calories In Vs. Calories Out

We've heard it all before. Weight loss is just a matter of "calories in vs. calories out" and the solution to everyone's weight problems are to just "eat less, exercise more."

While I generally agree the solutions to many health issues are simpler than some people make them out to be, sometimes they're not *that* simple. Yes, drastically reducing calories will often result in weight loss - for a period of time. But calories are merely one part of the equation. And prolonged calorie restriction may result in long term metabolic damage and nutritional deficiency if not done properly.

I've taken issue with the calories in vs. calories out mantra not because it is downright wrong, but because it is simply **incomplete**. Though there are some whose knowledge and work I admire, like Dave Asprey, who flat out disagree with the focus on calories. Dave has gone so far as to demonstrate one can lose fat by increasing calorie intake to 4,500 calories per day (2,000 above maintenance), eating entire sticks of butter, and not exercising. See: bulletproofexec.com/nutritional-fundamentalism-why-even-resolute-dieters-often-fail-nytimes-com

For me, "eat less, exercise more" is simply not the entire picture. I would hope it's obvious that eating a diet that consists purely of doughnuts and soft drinks, even if its low calorie, will not result in optimal health, fitness, and body composition regardless of its impact on body weight.

The body is complex and weight regulation is dependent on many interlinking factors such as hormones, genetics, inflammation, sleep, stress, toxin exposure, hormone receptor sensitivity, nutritional status, protein/fat/carbohydrate ratios and sources, timing of food intake, gut microflora, exercise type and intensity, amount of muscle mass, environmental temperature, etc.

But before you start to feel overwhelmed or hopeless because you think you may have trouble with one or more (or all) of these issues, realize that the solutions/fixes are often pretty simple (though not necessarily easy). Many times, it's just one or two things a person needs to change like getting more sleep and reducing excess sugar intake that fixes a lot of stuff all at once. In fact, by following all of the tips laid out in this guide, you'll address the root cause of the vast majority of health and weight issues whether you realize how it's happening or not.

For many people, it's simply a matter of "eat less junk, eat *more* nutritious food, and exercise properly for your specific goals." For more complex medical conditions, of course you should see a specialist.

The "hidden" sources of weight gain that are woefully left out in particular are: inflammation, stress management, and high toxins in the diet.

Inflammation can largely be reduced by grounding/earthing (see earthing.com), fish oil supplementation, reducing intake of oxidized vegetable oils and trans-fats, utilizing healthy spices like turmeric, and other healthy lifestyle actions.

Managing stress and negative emotions is covered in depth earlier in this guide.

Eating a low toxin diet is more difficult as many foods, even health foods, contain toxins when not properly prepared. But a good rule of thumb is to purchase organic food, preferably locally grown, and limit high toxin foods like non-organic corn, produce with a lot of pesticides, and poor quality meats. Also, see the section on detoxifying which provides additional measures for reducing toxin load on the body.

www.bulletproofexec.com/remove-toxins

www.bulletproofexec.com/not-the-calories-stupid-reply-to-time-magazine

20: Organic Quality Food At A Discount

It can be tough to genuinely want to eat the highest quality organic foods but have a limited budget. Organic food, particularly when it comes to organic and grass-fed meats, can end up being as much as 2-3 times as expensive as conventional food.

I should point out a reason for this is that the government subsidizes certain foods, and the reason "junk food" is so cheap is that it has been made cheaper for farmers to grow crops like corn and soy. Another reason is that organic produce is more likely to have crop loss due to insects.

But a big reason why organic can sometimes be more expensive is that the process of becoming certified organic can be more costly than what some farmers can afford to pay, even if their food would otherwise meet organic standards. This means that, with the right shopping techniques, you can purchase "organic quality" food at similar to conventional prices.

A great method for doing this is to shop locally at farmer's markets, buy direct from farmers, and to utilize Community Supported Agriculture programs (CSA). Find local farmers and CSA programs in your area by visiting localharvest.org.

Oftentimes, there are heavy discounts for food that is purchased in bulk and for joining monthly "membership" programs with local farms. You can also find local farmer's markets and get in contact with local farms directly. This allows you to talk to the farmers, learn about how they grow their food, and work out good deals on food that may be as good or better than certified organic food, even if they can't officially label their food "organic."

Another method I often use is to simply shop online for organic food.

BarryFarm.com is one of my favorite online stores along with

SunOrganicFarm.com

Discount grass-fed beef can be purchased at alderspring.com/store.

You can also find a local supplier of quality meat by visiting EatWild.com/products/index.html.

Slow Food is another company dedicated to helping people find high quality local produce. Go to the Local Chapters section at SlowFoodUsa.org.

21: Why You Should Break The Rules

Does it ever feel like there are a ton of "rules" when it comes to how to eat to get fit?

Things like:

"Don't eat carbohydrates (or anything) after 7pm."

"Eat 4-6 small meals a day."

"Eat a big breakfast."

"Get XYZ amount of protein, carbohydrates, and fats every day."

And the list goes on.

The problem is, some people get so caught up in trying to live by all of these rules, they lose sight of the big picture. It also creates a belief system that there is only one way to reach a goal.

Here's a secret, one of the most effective ways to burn fat and get in great shape is to eat most of your carbohydrates later at night. It's called "Carb Backloading" from carbbackloading.com

And did you know a lot of people gain more muscle and lose more fat by fasting and eating less frequently? Intermittent fasting, particularly the leangains.com approach, has gained a lot of popularity for going against the dogma of needing to eat 6 small meals a day by getting great results with 2-3 meals in an eight hour feeding window.

But my point is not to sell you on these approaches. Some people, in particular women, often do notice better results with smaller and more frequent meals. And it's certainly possible to stay slim easier by eating most of one's carbohydrates in a big breakfast and not eating after 7pm.

The point to all of this is to realize that all of these so called "rules" are rarely absolutes. A lot of times, they're effective simply because a person *believes* they're effective. And that's ok too. There's nothing wrong with utilizing a bit of the placebo effect (mind over matter) to one's advantage.

What I am pretty certain of however is that getting stressed out and becoming neurotic about the tiniest details while losing sight of the big picture *is* detrimental. Following strict rules and routines has its benefits for people who tend to be lax. It helps develop a certain level of discipline and creates structure. This kind of thinking is also essential for competitive bodybuilders, fitness models, and athletes, but it's rarely *necessary* for the average person.

To have the greatest effectiveness, one must be flexible. Bruce Lee puts it like this, "obey the principles without being bound by them."

This means for those who tend to be unstructured, having a few rules in place is just what they need... for a period of time. But once that discipline is developed, I've found a great benefit by breaking the rules, if even only for a period of time, just to prove to myself that the world will not end.

For instance, it was very freeing to know I didn't "have to" eat 6 small meals a day to stay in great shape which was what I was originally told. I also have found that for myself, 2-3 meals a day is a little on the low side and I do better with around 4 meals a day. But no matter what, the body will adapt to either approach to varying degrees.

By going to each extreme and not being attached to thinking I "have to" do anything in particular, I'm able to find what works best for me and continually adapt to my current circumstances. This also allows me to switch things up when what worked best for me a year ago or even yesterday might not still work best for me today. In other words, I obey the principles without being bound by them. I encourage you to do the same.

22: The Incredible Superfood You'll Love To Eat

There was a food so prized by the Aztecs, they considered it to be worth more than gold and even used it as a currency. Its name means "food of the gods" and it was especially prized for its ability to provide all day energy.

This food is one of the highest sources of antioxidants among any known food. Antioxidants provide protection against oxidation. Oxidation is the same process as "rusting" on metal, only it also happens inside your body resulting in aging and degeneration. The wrinkles around a smoker's mouth are a visible sign of oxidation's effects on a particular part of the body.

This food is among the highest sources of magnesium of any food, and magnesium is a big mineral deficiency in our modern society.

It's one of the only foods to contain neurotransmitters and hormone precursors. It helps boost serotonin which can fight off depression as well as anandamide which is the "bliss" hormone. It is one of only two foods to contain phenylethylamine which is the "love" chemical associated with the feelings of being in love.

This food is none other than the source of all chocolate, the cacao bean.

It wasn't until the addition of processed sugar and processing of the cacao that we end up with the chocolate treats that we typically think of as unhealthy. You may have heard of studies showing the health benefits of dark chocolate, and that's because it contains less sugar and fat and more of the anti-aging and health promoting cacao.

When I discovered this, I wondered, could it be that so many people instinctively crave chocolate because, in its raw form, it is one of the greatest health foods we've ever discovered as mankind? Knowing what I know about food cravings, I think this is very possible. Sometimes people crave something because their body knows that food will provide certain missing elements such as minerals, antioxidants, and mood boosters that are desparately needed.

I recommend getting as close to a pure raw cacao as possible. Some do not enjoy the bitter taste of raw cacao because they're so used to the highly processed conventional chocolate. I've found that I was able to develop not just a tolerance, but a *love* for raw cacao fairly quickly by doing just a few things.

The first is to gradually move to eating darker chocolates. Yes, you can eat chocolate and be healthy! Like coffee and other bitter foods, a person can readily adapt to the flavor if they gradually introduce it. Bitter foods are very important for health and are rarely consumed in the typical Western diet. I actually prefer the taste of dark chocolate now over lighter chocolates.

As a tolerance for bitter foods develops, one can then start to incorporate raw cacao with a healthier sweetener such as honey or stevia. It also makes an excellent addition to a smoothie where it can be used as a flavor enhancer. Cacao is also unique in that it can be used as a "driver" to aid in the absorption and taste of other herbs such as medicinal mushrooms.

One of my favorite ways to eat raw cacao is to melt some cacao butter in hot water or almond milk with a little cinnamon and raw honey to make a hot chocolate.

For more information on cacao and chocolate, check out:

amazon.com/Naked-Chocolate-Astonishing-Worlds-Greatest/dp/1556437315

thebestdayever.com/news/podcast/podcast-74-the-real-deal-on-cacao

longevitywarehouse.com - Where I find the best raw cacao.

23: Are Healthy Foods Hurting Your Body?

There are several reasons why I don't recommend a one-size-fits-all diet plan. And one of those reasons is because there are many foods that can be genuinely healthy, but be absolutely terrible for certain people.

I'm not talking about what foods are "always" bad for a certain body type, genetic profile, or even fitness goals. I'm talking about an issue that, while gaining more popularity, is something the vast majority of the population never even considers.

That issue is food intolerances.

Gluten (found in wheat, rye, barley, and some other grains), casein and lactose (found in milk products), soy, and eggs are extremely common intolerances. Intolerances to things like gluten in particular can cause damage to the digestive system resulting in inflammation.

What many people don't realize is that an intolerance can develop in individuals who, at one point, could handle the foods just fine. So just because a person does fine eating eggs every single day for a few years on end doesn't mean they can't eventually develop an intolerance towards them.

Symptoms can include mucous build up, digestive upset, skin rashes, and numerous other symptoms which can be so subtle, a person may not even realize their symptoms until they stop eating the food. To make things trickier, the symptoms may be delayed by up to a day or more after eating the problem food.

One reason food intolerances may develop is that the body needs a variety of foods. Our ancestors would have eaten different produce based on the season and different meats depending on what they were able to hunt for the day. We also need a variety of nutrients that no one particular food can meet, outside of perhaps just a few exceptional superfoods.

While there are certain foods that are fine to consume on a near daily basis, particularly those that lack protein (allergies are reactions to proteins), it's a good practice to rotate the foods you eat.

For some, this could mean switching up the foods you eat each day. For others, it could simply mean if you've been relying on a particular type of food for a while, such as chicken for protein, to switch it up for a while to something like fish.

If you suspect a food intolerance, try eliminating the most common problem foods for a while such as dairy, wheat, nuts, and soy for a couple weeks. Then gradually reintroduce foods to see how your body responds. You can also see a qualified specialist to get a proper elimination diet and testing.

24: Simple Substitutions For Healthier Food

Does eating healthier mean giving up your favorite comfort foods and flavors?

Not necessarily. With a few simple substitutions, you can eliminate the foods that promote fat gain and poor health and replace them with better alternatives that not only taste great, but actually enhance your health and fat loss efforts!

Sugar Substitutes

- Stevia - Stevia is the most popular of the "natural" non-sugar sweeteners. It is versatile and can be used for any application in which sugar is called for. It is available in both liquid (ideal for adding to beverages) and powder (ideal for baking) form.

- Xylitol - Xylitol is a naturally occurring sugar alcohol that is found in many fruits and vegetables. It does provide 2/3 as many calories as sugar, but without the downside of being too quickly absorbed. It can also help fight dental bacteria and promote fresh breathe!

- Raw Honey - Honey is very sweet as it is a natural source of sugar, including fructose. But before the sugar scares you off, realize that research has shown that when feeding rats sugar and honey, sugar resulted in a negative effect on triglycerides and oxidation while honey didn't have these negative effects. Not to mention honey has been used for thousands of years as a health food. It is filled with beneficial enzymes and minerals making it a nutritious sweetener rather than a source of empty calories like refined sugar. I suggest getting a local raw honey as well which can build tolerance towards local allergens. Despite its relative safety, it should still be consumed in moderation and limited by those with sugar sensitivities.

- Unsulphured Blackstrap Molasses - While blackstrap molasses isn't the sweetest, it is actually a health food that was often used for its healing qualities. It is filled with all the beneficial minerals that are stripped out of refined sugar and can even be used as an inexpensive mineral supplement.

Regular Salt Substitutes

Do you crave salty snacks? Perhaps that's because your body knows the health benefits of salt in its true, <u>mineral rich</u> form. While the best forms of sodium are likely vegetables such as celery and kelp, there may be some evidence that cutting back on salt isn't the answer to better health. Some studies have shown that salt is not only a non-issue for blood pressure except for a small fraction of individuals, but cutting back on it can increase the likelihood of death!

I believe that using an *unrefined* salt is not only an acceptable substitute for regular salt, but can actually be healthy and useful for individuals wishing to improve adrenal function and restore trace minerals almost everyone is deficient in. Some salts, like Dead Sea Salts, are rich in potassium, magnesium, and calcium in addition to their sodium content.

Good salts are any unrefined salts such as:

- Himalayan Salt
- Dead Sea Salt
- Celtic Sea Salt

Better Oil Substitutes

One of the worst things to ingest are the highly unnatural and refined vegetable oils like canola and soy oil. Even worse are the trans-fats (anything that reads partially-hyrogenated) common in processed snacks and baked goods. But even healthier oils like olive oil can be damaged and rendered rancid when cooking.

So what can you do if you have a recipe that calls for heavy amounts of oil? Utilize these healthier oils for your cooking and general health needs:

- Coconut Oil – Great for fat loss and very heat stable. High in beneficial a type of saturated fat called medium chain triglycerides that can actually help burn body fat!

- Palm Oil – Rich in vitamin E and antioxidants. Safe for high temperature cooking.

- Macadamia Oil – Excellent for high temperature cooking and a great source of Omega 7 fatty acids. Omega 7 (Palmitoleic Acid) has many benefits including aiding the digestive track and it is a powerful antioxidant.

- Applesauce – While not an oil, applesauce can be used in exchange for oils in baked good recipes in a 1:1 ratio. For instance, 1 cup of applesauce can replace 1 cup of vegetable oil.

Grain Substitutes

If you're striving to reduce your intake of gluten or grains, then it can be a challenge to find a suitable flour replacement. Here are some good flour alternatives:

- Almond flour – Healthy fats and a rich flavor. Good for breads.

- Buckwheat Flour – High in protein and rich in D-Chiro-Inositol which helps blood sugar balance.

- Zucchini – Can be used to replace noodles for pasta recipes.

- Coconut Flour – Typically mixed with other flours, coconut flour is high in fiber.

- Quinoa – A tasty dish that is cooked up similar to rice. Rich in protein and nutrients. As it has gained popularity, there are some companies that make quinoa noodles and other wheat substitutes with quinoa.

Dairy Substitutes

I want to point out that cultured dairy like kefir and raw dairy may still be tolerated well by those otherwise sensitive to conventional dairy products. This is because the probiotics present in these foods help pre-digest the lactose and casein. Even for the general population I recommend utilizing cultured dairy far more than non-cultured dairy.

Many people when looking to get away from dairy turn to soy milk and soy products. I do NOT recommend this as these soy products may have negative effects on hormones. While a little bit of organic soy won't hurt every now and then, daily consumption isn't suggest. Instead, try some of these better dairy alternatives.

- Hemp Milk
- Coconut Milk
- Almond Milk
- Oat Milk

25: A Missing Link To Good Health

Researchers have found an interesting difference in the bodies of some lean vs. obese people, and it's not that they have different genes. It's something that most people never even think about, but this one thing plays a significant role in your health, hormone levels, and immune system function.

That one thing is the colony of beneficial bacteria you have living in your gut.

The reason why gut bacteria may play a role in obesity is because more and more research shows they play a role in just about *everything* in your body from hormone levels, depression and mood, immune function, digestion, vitamin production and absorption, and more. There are actually about ten times as many bacteria in your gut as there are cells in your body!

In other words, they're kind of a big deal.

The problem is that because of stress, antibiotics, and a diet lacking in cultured foods, most people have an imbalance in their gut bacteria resulting in an overgrowth of harmful bacteria and fungi. The "good guy" bacteria that are supposed to be protecting you are missing, and no amount of healthy foods and lifestyle intervention can make up for their absence.

This is why increasing your intake of probiotics is so important. But before you think that eating a little bit of yogurt is going to take care of you, realize that most store bought yogurt has minimal intact probiotics. To complicate things even more, there's between 500-1000 different species of probiotics in the human gut while foods and supplements may only have a few strains.

Scientists find that not all probiotic strains are created equal. For instance, there are many different strains of lactobacillus acidophilus which research shows has differing effects depending on which strain is ingested. So just because a person took something with "acidophilus" and didn't notice any benefits, doesn't mean a different strain of acidophilus like DDS-1 couldn't be highly beneficial.

It appears that the best protection is to avoid pharmaceutical antibiotics whenever they're not necessary as they will kill the healthy bacteria along with the bad. Unfortunately, for many people the damage has been done.

The most effective option for probiotic restoration is not something many people would consider, and that's fecal transplants. Literally taking feces from one healthy individual and putting it into someone else to recolonize the gut. While this is, to the best of my knowledge, one of the most effective means we currently have of effectively restoring proper gut bacteria, it is a lesser known and little practiced technique for probably a variety of reasons unrelated to its effectiveness.

Regardless of whether or not one wants to go that far, it's very good to include cultured foods like **raw** sauerkraut, kimchi, and kefir into one's diet which you can make yourself at home with a starter kit from bodyecology.com. You may also find these foods at farmer's markets and health food stores, albeit they're usually much more expensive than what you can make yourself.

Finally, probiotic supplements can be used to fill in the gaps and target certain health issues like poor digestion. But the number of living bacteria per capsule is much smaller than in cultured foods and may not repopulate the gut as readily as food based probiotics like kefir and sauerkraut.

Here are some of the best probiotic supplements out there. While there are many good products out there, these are some of the best for various needs.

- **Saccharomyces Boulardii**: This is an important probiotic to take because it stimulates sIgA production. sIgA is needed for proper signaling to the immune system which bacteria are currently in our gut. To make a long story short, this enhances the benefits of *all* the other probiotics you will take. Without adequate sIgA signaling however, the probiotics won't do their job as well. Read more about this at: nutricology.com/infocus/pdfletters/InFocus_2009Oct_Probiotics.pdf

- **Lactobacillus GG**: Lactobacillus GG (brand name Culturelle) is one of the most researched and time-tested strains of bacteria with over 400 studies done on it. It's well noted for its immune enhancing effects, improvement of digestion, and its ability to successfully survive the digestive track intact to colonize the gut. It has been shown to aid in fighting infection and improve the skin with conditions like eczema. It is my number #1 recommendation when starting probiotics as there are few if any that can match the research backing it has.

- **Bifantis – Bifidobacterium infantis**: Bifantis (brand name Align) is well-known for its benefits on digestion. It is great for those suffering from irritable bowel syndrome. This is typically the first probiotic to recommend for digestive issues.

- **L. Acidophilus Strain DDS-1**: The DDS-1 strain is a highly researched strain of L. Acidophilus that is of human origin. This means it works well within the human body and can tolerate transition through the digestive track. Like other strains, research has shown it is extremely beneficial for gut-health as well as enhancing the immune system.

- **Jarro-Dophilus EPS**: The #1 probiotic blend in the US.

- **Natren Trinity**: Natren is also the only company I've seen to have the Malytho superstrain of Bifidobacterium bifidum.

Wondering which probiotic to take? I suggest using a single strain to begin with and assess how you feel. This could be Saccharomyces to begin with, then trying Culturelle, DDS-1, and/or Align one at a time to see how you feel on each. Eventually, you can try moving on to a blend. Several good brands for probiotic blends also include Custom Probiotics, New Chapter, and Dr. Ohhira's.

Just because one probiotic product doesn't work well for you, doesn't mean another one couldn't be the "missing link" you've been looking for. That being said, sometimes people don't respond well to any probiotics. This could be a sign of gut damage and inflammation. Glut Immune (a type of Glutamine) and N-Aceytl Glucosamine are two of the most powerful things I am aware of for repairing the digestive track.

For more information on the benefits of probiotics and cultured foods, I highly suggest the book "The Body Ecology Diet" by Donna Gates. It is one of the best diet books I've ever read.

26: One Trick To Go From Dull To Delectable

There's one big trade-off I used to make when cooking meals in a hurry, and that was oftentimes I would sacrifice taste for convenience.

This was particularly an issue when I first got into healthy eating. I was "hardcore" in my motivation to get fit, so I would force down dry and bland chicken breasts, raw broccoli, and plain rice all in order to reach my fitness goals. I had the attitude that if it tastes good, it can't be good for me.

Since then, I have not only discovered a simple trick that makes the most boring meals taste amazing, but it actually *enhances* the nutrition content for additional health benefits. (Hint: It's not just adding a few dried spices)

My favorite method of kicking up the taste and health of foods is to make a few special homemade sauces that I can prepare in bulk and keep in my refrigerator. I usually just blend the ingredients in a mini-blender, but some can be made in a mixing bowl.

There are literally endless options here based on your unique tastes and the type of dish, but I've found a few "go-to" sauces that work with a lot of meals. Here are just a couple of my favorites:

Guacamole: I take a healthier organic salsa bought from the store (note: salsa is a pretty good condiment all by itself for those who don't want to make anything), and blend it with fresh avocado in a mini-blender. I may also throw in one clove of fresh garlic to kick up the taste.

Salsa: Although finding healthier store bought varieties of salsa isn't terribly difficult, making your own is a simple option as well. Combine tomatoes (optionally cooked), onions, peppers, cayenne, chiles, and lime juice. Cilantro is a great addition for its powerful detoxification effects and the flavor

Onion Cream: I like using coconut milk (the kind found in a can) for this recipe to get in the healthy fats from coconut. Blend 8oz of canned unsweetened coconut milk (or Greek yogurt) with 1

large onion. Add ½ teaspoon of salt, ½ teaspoon garlic powder, and ½ teaspoon of pepper. May add other spices to taste.

Curry Sauce: Blend one can of unsweetened coconut milk with 2 tablespoons of curry powder. May optionally add 1 teaspoon cayenne pepper for a spicier curry. I usually add this to recipes before cooking.

Pumpkin Sauce: Combine 8oz of pumpkin, ½ cup almond milk, 1 clove garlic, 1 teaspoon of pumpkin pie spice, and 1 tablespoon honey.

If you want some recipes that are healthy and taste great, check out these resources:

youtube.com/user/leanbodylifestyle and the new channel youtube.com/user/michaelkoryfitness are both great sources for tasty and healthy recipes for fitness minded individuals.

bodybuilding.com/fun/bbmainnut/food-recipes.html – has tons of great healthy recipes

http://cookinglight.com has a variety of lower calorie recipes.

While not strictly health, you can visit yummly.com to find a variety of recipes, and simply utilize some of the safe substitutions to enhance the health factor of the recipes you find.

27: Not So Healthy "Health Foods"

I see a lot of people struggling because they believe they're eating a "healthy" diet, but are in actuality kidding themselves. While there's endless debate as to what is or isn't healthy, there are a few things that are generally agreed upon as not ideal for maximum fat loss and longevity.

The caveat I want to make before getting into this is that it is highly debatable as to how "bad" any particular food really is. Really, just about anything can be enjoyed in moderation without overly negative consequences. The point here is to make note of the things that people "trick" themselves into believing they can eat as much as they want to and not have any drawbacks.

The simplest diet advice comes from Jack Lalane who says "if man made it, don't eat it." While I wouldn't take this *too* literally, it does have a lot of truth when it comes to the highly processed garbage a lot of people are eating mistakenly believing it to be healthy.

Here are a few common things people eat when trying to eat healthier that may not be such a good idea:

- **Salad Dressings** – While most people don't consider the salad dressings to be what makes a salad healthy, some people inadvertently think their salad is helping them get fit despite drenching it with terrible dressings. Most conventional salad dressings are filled with poor vegetable oils like soy or canola oil and/or tons of sugar. A salad topped these dressings can be just as fattening as many of the foods people are replacing with the salads. Opt instead for olive oil and vinegar, one of the few healthy salad dressings made without oils/sweeteners/perservatives, or make your own dressing with apple cider vinegar and cayenne pepper. Or, simply utilize the 60 second salad recipe I provide here: excuseproof.com/salad

- **Conventional Yogurt** – While homemade yogurt, or even better yogurt from raw milk from a local farm, can be very nutritious, most of the stuff bought at stores is far from being a health food. They're typically filled with tons of sugar or artificial sweeteners. I suggest using either a Greek yogurt, or purchasing a good quality organic plain yogurt (or even better kefir) and adding in your own fresh berries and/or honey.

- **Whole Wheat Breads And Muffins** – Wheat isn't that much of a health food to begin with, so having something "whole wheat" doesn't make it all that much better. While I don't say everyone needs to avoid wheat or gluten, many people may be better off *reducing* it in their diet. These foods are also usually filled with added sugar, oils, and artificial ingredients not typically found in homemade bread. A better alternative is to use a sprouted grain bread like Ezekial makes if you still want wheat, or try a healthier organic rice, potato, or almond bread.

- **Diet Soft Drinks** – Some claim the artificial sweeteners in diet soft drinks are worse than the sugar they're replacing. There does seem to be evidence that they indirectly lead to weight gain. I can't say one way or another whether artificial sweeteners are that bad, but I do know every diet soft drink consumed is taking the place of something healthier like pure water, tea, or even coffee (which has its health benefits). While likely fine in moderation as most things are, I would advise not overdoing it with the diet drinks.

- **Conventional Soy** – Conventional (as opposed to organic) soy is typically genetically modified which poses questions about the health and safety of it. All soy is also high in phytoestrogens which experts debate about their potential health consequences. Some say they're beneficial, others say they're harmful. I'd rather err on the side of safety and keep soy intake to a minimum and exclusively from occasionally eaten organic, whole food sources rather than the highly processed soy burgers, soy milks, soy cheeses, soy proteins, etc.

28: Teas For Any Of Your Needs

Tea is one of the most widely consumed beverages in the world. All the various "true" teas like black, green, oolong, and white tea provide a rich source of antioxidants, cancer fighting compounds, and seem to aid in just about every health condition.

As great as these teas are, there are also a lot of herbal teas out there filled with health promoting and fat burning qualities. Let's take a look at some of the best teas out there:

Green Tea: Green tea is rich in a compound called EGCG that has shown benefits for protecting against cancer, oxidative stress, heart disease, and is used to aid in fat loss.

White Tea: White tea has the highest antioxidant levels of all the true teas.

Gynostemma Tea: Gynostemma is an herb that has many benefits similar to ginseng in that it helps balance the body's systems and build up defense against stress. Some of the longest lived people in China were found to drink gynostemma tea on a regular basis. It is caffeine free. My preferred source is Spring Dragon Longevity Tea from Dragon Herbs. See: dragonherbs.com/prodinfo.asp?number=601

Yerba Matte Tea: Yerba matte is very similar to green tea in that it is often drank to boost energy, without burning you out. It also is traditionally drank as a weight loss aid and is even higher in antioxidants than green tea.

Rooibos Tea: Like other teas, rooibos is very high in antioxidants, including antioxidants that can't be found in any other tea, but it is free from caffeine.

Chamomile Tea: Chamomile is a popular night time tea because of its ability to relax the nerves and help one wind down. But its benefits go even further to reducing inflammation, boosting the immune system, and protecting against diabetes.

Horsetail and Nettle Tea: This combination is the ideal formula for improving bone health. These plants contain high amounts of silica (and magnesium) which may be even more important than calcium for building strong bones.

Pau d'Arco and Cat's Claw (Una De Gato): These herbs from the Amazon rainforest are two of the most powerful anti-fungal, anti-viral, and anti-bacterial herbs out there. People suffering from fungal/yeast infections as well as health complications from various bacterial and viral infections (or simply wishing to prevent infection and stay healthy) have noticed great benefit from utilizing multiple cups of these teas daily.

Of course, just about any medicinal herb can be made into a "tea." Here are a few good sources of healthy herbal teas to meet your specific health needs:

dragonherbs.com
traditionalmedicinals.com
longevitywarehouse.com

29: Healthy Meals On The Go In Seconds

What do you do when you have about 60 seconds to get a meal together, and maybe about another 60 seconds to actually eat that meal?

Well, besides the 60 second salad of course!

The answer for most people is to utilize a meal replacement that's either in powder or pre-mixed liquid form.

Typically these meal replacements are made with cheap proteins, some sugar and/or artificial sweeteners, and a bunch of low quality vitamins and minerals (not all vitamins and minerals are created equal) to give the illusion of being good for you.

While these are certainly convenient, and I've had my fair share of meal replacements, there's a couple problems with them.

One is, they're oftentimes not that healthy. Or at least, they're not as healthy as whole foods. Granted, you *can* find healthier meal replacements, but then they're often high priced and harder to find.

The other issue is, unless the meal replacement has an added fiber or appetite suppressing component (which some popular weight loss shakes do), they're often not very filling.

But what if there was a way to get the convenience of meal replacements, with the health benefits and appetite fulfillment of whole foods, all for a price that is reasonable for just about any budget?

I developed this strategy to meet all of those needs. And while meal replacements will never be as ideal as whole food meals, with a busy lifestyle, sometimes what is ideal must come secondary to what is practical.

What I do is start with an empty shaker bottle. I will add only powder ingredients. Since I keep a large jug of water bottle with me at all times (bonus tip: do the same), I'll simply add water when I'm ready to drink/eat.

I combine any of the following ingredients:

- **Protein Powder:** Hemp, Whey Concentrate, Rice, Pea, and/or Micellar Casein (avoid soy)

- **Fiber:** Ground flax seed, ground chia seed, coconut flour

- **Flavor:** Cacao powder, carob powder, dried vanilla, instant coffee

- **Healthy Fats:** Almond meal, coconut flour, MCT powder

- **Healthy Carbs:** Oat flour or ground oatmeal flakes, brown rice flour

- **Vitamins/Minerals/Nutrition/Superfood:** Greens blend such as Vitamineral Green, Spirulina, Chlorella, Moringa, Camu Camu, Noni powder, Mangosteen powder, Etc.

For example, I could put whey protein, almond flour, and some shredded oats (rolled oats processed in a coffee grinder) into an empty shaker cup. I can optionally add in other beneficial things like greens and herbal powders to kick up the micronutrients. Then whenever I'm ready to eat, I add some water to the shaker cup, shake, and then enjoy a satisfying meal that will keep my appetite satisfied for hours and provide some healthy whole food nutrition all at once.

I purchase raw ingredients from truenutrition.com at wholesale prices. They also allow you to custom make your own meal replacement shakes using some healthier proteins, carbohydrates, and fats with your own desired flavor and sweetener. Use discount code DKD714 to save on your order.

30: Quick Fix Snacks Foods That Won't Add Fat

I've talked to many people who've felt like being busy was the biggest obstacle to getting and staying fit. The truth is however, there are many healthy and fit people that are crazy busy. One of the things busy fit people know is which foods are ideal for snacking on and taking on the go.

Here are some of the simplest snacks you can eat that take little to no preparation.

Fruits: This is stating the obvious, but apples, bananas, peaches, grapes, and other fruits are portable and convenient. Be careful with dried fruit however as they can be very high in sugar.

Nuts: Nuts are very nutritionally rich foods and provide healthy fats and protein. They are good for a low carbohydrate snack, but similar to dried fruit, they can be easy to overeat. Avoid nuts that contain large amounts of unnatural flavorings, oils, etc and instead opt for raw nuts or dry roasted nuts. Even better, soak raw nuts overnight, then let them dry to sprout them for even better nutrition and digestion.

If plain nuts are too bland for your taste, I like to take a small mason jar or plastic bag, fill it with slivered almonds (any nut is fine), and combine with spices such as a good seasoning mix, garlic powder, cayenne pepper, and whatever else I'd like. If need be, I can add a little olive oil or coconut oil so the spices stick. I then shake up the container and can take it with me on the go for a quick and easy spicy nuts treat.

Vegetables: Like raw fruits and nuts, raw vegetables are about as simple and easy as it gets when it comes to quick food options. Things like celery (may add almond or nut butters), carrot slices, cherry tomatoes, cucumber, and snap peas can all be eaten on their own or combined in a large container (prepare in bulk) and stored ready to be put in a smaller container to for on the go. I also enjoy keeping a large container of cultured vegetables in the refrigerator to snack on any time with some salsa.

Goji Berries: Not only do goji berries make a convenient and tasty snack, but they are arguably one of the best foods/herbs in the world for anti-aging. Their importance for the tonic (balancing) effects they have on health go back thousands of years in Chinese medicine. Only an ounce or two a day is needed for the benefits making them fairly economical at about $1 a day. Dragon Herbs sell the best quality Goji berries.

Cacao Nibs: Raw cacao provides all the health benefits of chocolate without the downsides or "guilt." If straight raw cacao nibs are too bitter, my suggestion would be to include nibs in a "trail mix" with some sweet fruit like raisins. You can also spice them up with some cinnamon. Keep in mind cacao is a powerful food and it's possible to either eat too much or find you have a sensitivity to it all together. Some people do not handle cacao well and it's better to listen to your body.

Rice Cakes: Brown rice cakes and flavored rice cakes are some of my favorite snacks as they are tasty, gluten-free, and affordable. Go for the kind that don't add much sweetener. Lundberg's rice cake products, both organic and regular, are excellent. I realize some may say rice cakes are not ideal for fat loss, but I don't believe anyone got too fat on brown rice if they're physically active. As a bonus tip, get the kind with cinnamon as cinnamon helps blood sugar balance and in turn aids in fat loss.

Pickles: Low in calories, tart, and filling. Pickles make a great snack when a person wants something salty and crunchy to snack on without packing on the pounds.

Dried Olives: Full of beneficial fats and portable.

Hard Boiled Eggs: Portable protein on the go. Add a bit of garlic powder, salt, and pepper to spice these up.

Homemade Protein Bars: Making your own healthy bars is easy. There are a variety of recipes online and you can start with these healthy ones:

- bodybuilding.com/fun/diy-protein-bars-healthy-bars-in-5-easy-steps.html
- healthygreenkitchen.com/homemade-protein-bars.html
- quicheaweek.wordpress.com/2012/10/07/protein-bars-no-bake-and-baked-versions
- askmen.com/sports/foodcourt_200/244_protein-bar-recipes.html

31: The Nutrients You're Likely Lacking

The stressful lifestyles and poor diets of modern day times makes it virtually impossible to get all the nutrients a person needs to thrive and achieve optimal health. And if you think taking a multivitamin has your nutritional needs covered, chances are, it won't be nearly enough.

One reason for this is that most typical multivitamins are high in isolated vitamins and minerals that aren't as well absorbed and utilized by the body as when the vitamins and minerals come from whole foods. The other reason is that many people have nutritional deficiencies so severe, they need to take heavy doses of certain nutrients just to get to baseline.

The ideal way to determine what you need is through testing. I recommend spectracell.com to test your vitamin and mineral status. Then, utilize foods rich in the missing nutrients followed by supplementation with quality vitamin and mineral supplements only if needed.

But even without testing, there's almost a guarantee that unless you've proactively taken steps to get these nutrients, you will likely be deficient.

Vitamin D: Vitamin D is produced by the body after being exposed to the sun. It is highly cancer protective and needed for optimal bone health. The benefits could go on for the rest of this book, so I'll simply say make sure you get enough through either moderate sun exposure if you live in a sunny area (hard to do) and/or supplementation with vitamin D3 of 1000IU per 25 pounds of body weight per day. A blood test is the most accurate way to determine your specific needs.

Magnesium: Magnesium is a common mineral deficiency resulting in trouble sleeping, anxiety, fatigue, and poor bone health. Cacao, greens, and many nuts are rich in magnesium. Taking 500-1000 mg of a chelated magnesium and/or using magnesium oil is recommended.

Zinc: Another common deficiency, zing is necessary for proper hormone production and immune system health. Ant extract (yes, an extract made from bugs), pumpkin seeds, beef, oysters, and cacao are good sources. If supplementing with higher doses of zinc, you may wish to include a natural source of copper as well because too much zinc can deplete copper. Cacao is a good source of both zinc and copper.

Omega 3: Omega 3 levels are very low among the general population including even health conscious vegans who don't consume fish products. Adequate omega 3 levels is necessary for creating a proper cell membrane and keeping inflammation low. Fish oil is the ideal source of EPA and DHA. Krill oil is acceptable, but it is often very expensive for the amounts of EPA and DHA it contains and doesn't have the same research backing it like fish oil does. Algae oil is a source of DHA for vegans. Suggested dose is 1-5 grams a day of fish oil.

32: The Only Herbs You'll Ever Need

In our modern times, we have grown accustomed to the idea of taking a specific medicine to treat a specific symptom. But this often leads to unwanted side effects as the medicines force the body to raise or lower things forcefully creating imbalance in the body.

For instance, many people address having low energy by taking a high dose of caffeine which does result in more energy, but then that energy comes crashing down as the body recovers.

What if there was an herb so powerful, and so "intelligent" if you will, that regardless of what health condition you have, it would go to work to fix exactly what *you* needed fixed **without** throwing anything else out of balance?

There exists such an herb, but it's not just a single herb. It's an entire classification of herbs which are called adaptogenic herbs, or tonic herbs in Chinese medicine. These herbs are so safe to take, they can be treated as food and used everyday.

A common example of this would be ginseng. A good quality, aged ginseng is high in dual directional sapponins. These sapponins can work wherever and however the body needs them most.

A good quality adaptogenic herb will raise what is low in the body, and lower what is raised. That means for people low in energy, an herb can be energizing. But people too high strung will be calmed down by the same herb. There's no worry these herbs won't be a good fit for you as they fit your needs.

Adaptogenic herbs are the most valued for their ability to gradually heal the body and promote longevity. They work in particular on helping the body cope with stress as these herbs themselves often grow in and adapt to harsh environments.

Outside of having good whole food nutrition, taking a good quality adaptogenic herb or herbal formula is virtually essential in our high stressed and toxic world. Here are a few of my favorites:

Chaga: Chaga is a medicinal mushroom that typically grows in cold environments like Siberia on birch trees. This is one of the most powerful and unique herbs for health a person can take. This is a powerful tonic for boosting the immune system, fighting cancer, and promoting longevity. If I could only supplement with one herb, it would be chaga.

Reishi: The only herb that can rival chaga. Reishi has shown incredible power in fighting cancer and modulating the immune system. If I could only take two herbs, it would be chaga and reishi.

Ashwagandha: Ashwagandha is an herb that has been shown to support the thyroid, adrenals, and reduce excess cortisol. It's also very affordable and is my #1 herb of choice for *everyone* to take, even those on a budget, as it only costs a few dollars a month.

Astragalus: Astragalus is a premiere herb for boosting the immune system, strengthening muscles, and enhancing the metabolism. A great choice for those wishing to prevent sickness.

Schizandra: One of the most balanced herbs, it nourishes every part of the body. Overtime, this will strengthen anything that could be deficient leading to radiant health.

Rhodiola: Grown in high altitudes, rhodiola is of particular significance for athletes and those wishing to increase oxygenation. It helps improve endurance and helps one adapt to high altitudes.

Cordyceps: Similar benefits as rhodiola, cordyceps has a powerful ability to increase endurance and VO2 max while also providing similar benefits as chaga, reishi, and other medicinal mushrooms.

Ginseng: The most common tonic herb in the world. There are a variety of ginsengs with slightly different qualities. American ginseng is considered to be the most balanced, and is heavily imported into China. Panax ginseng is generally considered to be a bit more energizing.

Goji Berries: Goji berries are not only a tasty snack, but they help boost growth hormone, improve mood, and boost levels of superoxide dismutase, one of the body's most powerful antioxidants.

There are of course a variety of other tonic and adaptogenic herbs which are all worthwhile. Taking a combination formula allows one to get the benefits of a multitude of these herbs. Talking to someone knowledgeable in herbalism may help guide you to the best tonic herbs for your unique circumstances.

My #1 pick regardless of budget is chaga which is still very affordable at $25 a bottle from Dragon Herbs. My pick for those on a budget is ashwagandha.

My favorite supplier of quality adaptogenic herbs and Chinese medicinal herbs are dragonherbs.com and jingherbs.com.

33: Avoiding Sickness With A Super Immune System

Getting sick sucks. But the immune system is responsible for a lot more than just warding off the flu. A strong and well functioning immune system is also what keeps cancer at bay. The body is also constantly defending itself against infections that, if unmanaged, can lead to skin problems, yeast infections, low energy, and degenerating health even if one doesn't have an overt "sickness."

But simply amplifying the immune response isn't always desirable. A strong immune response directed at the body itself in the form of an allergy is sometimes more harmful than pathogens.

What we want is a balanced immune system that responds effectively to pathogens without overreacting and attacking the body itself. This can be accomplished through something known as immune modulation, and it is one of the qualities of adaptogenic herbs like chaga, reishi, and astragalus which is why I recommend them so highly.

The basic steps to a proper functioning immune system are to eat a nutritious diet, minimize stress, and eat probiotic rich foods. But sometimes we need some extra support.

Here are some suggested products for a super immune system. Note that many of these products are best taken in moderate doses daily throughout the year to ensure constant good health. If taken after getting sick, they may help reduce the time and severity of infection, but won't necessarily stop sickness outright.

Natural Vitamin C: One of the most common things people turn to when they get sick is vitamin C. While vitamin C is important for the immune system, high doses of vitamin C in the form of supplemental ascorbic acid isn't ideal as it lacks other co-factors found in whole foods. Opt for a whole food source of vitamin C like Camu Camu berry either in addition to or instead of ascorbic acid.

6-Hour Colostrum: Colostrum is what a mother cow produces to feed her newborn calf shortly after birth. It is responsible for literally creating the immune system of the baby calf. Colostrum is unlike any other food in it that it contains 97 immune factors and 87 growth factors that can help rebuild a "broken" immune system when one takes it. The 6-Hour colostrum I recommend is collected within the first six hours of calving, and it is taken from from the excess produced so the baby calves still get their fair share making it ethically sound. Find it here: longevitywarehouse.com

Silver Hydrosol: Silver is one of the most powerful natural antibiotic products available. Many colloidal silver products are ineffective. Plus, improperly made silver products can cause an accumulation of silver in the body. But a high quality silver hydrosol is one of the most powerful and safe things a person can use internally or topically to kill off any infections. I suggest Argentyn 23 as in my research and personal use, it seems most effective without any risk of accumulation or toxicity with proper usage.

Pau d'Arco and Cat's Claw (Una De Gato): These can be taken in extract form for even more powerful infection fighting power. These are particularly useful when dealing with stubborn infections and fungal issues.

Adaptogenic Herbs: The various adaptogenic herbs will all work to keep the immune system functioning properly with the most notable being the various medicinal mushrooms as well as astragalus. Taking this as a regular part of your lifestyle will help prevent sickness and keep the immune system strong all year round.

Vitamin D: Necessary for numerous aspects of good health and in particular immune system function.

34: Be Pain Free Naturally

Besides diminishing quality of life, being in pain can make it difficult to exercise and stay physically active.

Over the years of studying nutrition, I've found there are a couple common, and not so common ways to heal and lubricate joints, rebuild tissue, and cut down on inflammation. There are also some pretty cool tricks for overcoming muscle soreness.

Here are a few of my favorite products for joint health and natural pain relief:

Cissus: Cissus Quadrangularis is an herb that is powerful for rebuilding joints and even has some benefits for fat loss and muscle gain. It is my go to supplement for rebuilding broken down tissue and surviving grueling weight training. USP Labs makes the best cissus product.

Celadrin: Celadrin is available as both a topical cream and supplement. This is a formula of oils that lubricate the joints for greater range of motion, reduced inflammation, and has no side effects.

Glucosamine and Chondroitin: The most common joint supplements for improving joint health. Worth trying, but I recommend trying Cissus and Celadrin if not finding relief from glucosamine.

Camu Camu: Very beneficial for arthritis relief and a great source of vitamin C.

Hydrolyzed Collagen: Reduces inflammation and enhances joint health. May be more effective than glucosamine.

Turmeric/Curcumin: Curcumin is the main active component of turmeric, a common spice used in curries. Curcumin is a natural anti-inflammatory and pain reliever with numerous health benefits. Supplementing with curcumin is a great way to reduce pain naturally while achieving a host of other health benefits. I also highly suggest including turmeric in your diet as much as possible as it also enhances fat loss, protects against cancer, and is a natural detoxifier.

Magnesium: Taking a bath in either Epsom salts (magnesium sulfate) or dead sea salts is a great way to relieve sore muscles. Magnesium oil may also be used on achy muscles to provide targeted relief.

Traumeel: A cream that can be used on sore muscles for relief.

35: A Fat That Burns Fat?

What if a type of fat we've been told our whole life was "evil" was actually the fat that can help you the most when it comes to burning fat, improving your heart health, and filling you with long lasting and sustainable energy?

This type of fat supports the adrenal glands and thyroid, has anti-viral, anti-fungal, and anti-bacterial effects, and can be utilized by cells for energy without requiring insulin.

This fat is none other than saturated fat, or more accurately a specific class of saturated fat known as medium chain triglycerides (MCT).

Medium chain triglycerides like lauric and caprylic acid, which are found in things like coconut and palm oil, provide all of these benefits and more. Of particular importance for fitness minded people is that when replacing some other fats in the diet with these, people tend to lose more fat while reporting more energy.

Bonus Tip: Coconut oil makes an excellent natural skin and hair moisturizer that won't clog pores.

A simple method of utilizing these in your diet is to include 1-3 tablespoons of coconut oil daily. Another more powerful option is to actually use a MCT oil at 1-3 tablespoons a day.

Dave Asprey of the Bulletproof Executive encourages people to combine MCT oil with coffee in the morning for sustained energy. www.bulletproofexec.com/bulletproof-coffee-recipe

Now that may seem like a lot of fat, but this fat is going to provide energy the body will burn up rather than store, encourage fat loss, and ideally be replacing less healthy fats like vegetable oils.

Another benefit of coconut oil and palm oil is that they're ideal cooking oils. Simply replacing vegetable oils, olive oil, margarine, or cooking sprays with these fats is a simple step to improve health and cut down on inflammation.

Coconut oil is solid at room temperature so you'll need to melt it if it is solidified. The unrefined coconut oils, which I recommend, can also can have a strong flavor by itself, but I've found it easy to mask when using in smoothies. It actually enhances the flavor of protein shakes by providing a richer and creamier texture.

Any virgin (preferably organic but not essential) coconut oil is fine and typically pretty affordable when ordered online from amazon.com. Higher quality coconut oil and other tropical oils can be purchased from tropicaltraditions.com where you'll also find a variety of coconut based recipes. The direct link to the recipes is freecoconutrecipes.com/index.htm.

36: What Fixes Thyroid Issues Naturally

The thyroid gland, which is responsible for producing hormones related to energy usage and metabolism, plays a big role in person's ability to lose or gain weight. Those with experiencing hypothyroidism (under-active thyroid) may find weight loss difficult while those with hyperthyroid (overactive thyroid) may find weight gain difficult.

A simple home test that can be done to determine thyroid function is something called the "Barnes" test. It is done by taking your temperature under the tongue first thing in the morning. 97.2 - 98.2 degrees fahrenheit (36.2 - 36.8 celsius) is considered normal. If you find your temperature falls below this, that may be a sign of under-active thyroid. Menstruating women should only take this test the 2nd or 3rd day after menstruation begins.

If you find your thyroid is over or under active, is there a way to bring the thyroid back into balance naturally?

Yes, but first you should always follow a doctor's advice. Luckily, many thyroid prescriptions are made from natural thyroid and are good options. What I want to share with you here is simply what I've learned from a few doctors who've had tremendous success in treating both overactive and under-active thyroid with some natural interventions.

Before anything else, realize that the thyroid will be affected by foods you eat. Vegetable oils like soy, canola, safflower, etc. are particularly bad for the thyroid as they're often oxidized as well as foods high in goitrogens like soy and lots of raw cruciferious vegetables like broccolli (which are fine in moderation and better when lightly cooked).

Also, things in the body do not work in isolation. Thyroid and adrenal issues often come hand in hand. I believe the safest course of action, for minor thyroid issues, is to use adaptogenic herbs to gradually bring the body back into balance. Ashwagandha (Sensoril Extract) is particularly useful for helping both the thyroid and adrenals rebalance while reducing excess cortisol.

Looking at the thyroid, the most common mineral that comes to mind is iodine. Iodine is particularly important for the thyroid, but it also plays a role in other areas of the body and may be cancer protective. Conventional thinking says that iodine deficiency is rare due to iodized salt, and that too much iodine is harmful and leads to the thyroid problems.

The work of Dr. David Brownstein and Dr. Guy Abraham have shown that supplementing with higher doses of iodine is not only safe, but very effective in treating many thyroid conditions including *both* over and under active thyroid. Many Asian countries take in significant quantities of iodine through sea vegetables and maintain great health and thyroid function. This seems to indicate that whole food sources of organic kelp and dulse may be some of the best protection for the thyroid, and these foods are pretty much completely absent in the Western diet.

High doses of supplemental iodine like Lugol's iodine is often used in treatment, and this may be ok but is a little more risky as it's easier to overdo it and find yourself detoxing. The reason for detoxing is that bromide accumulation occurs in the body in the absence of adequate iodine, and when iodine levels are restored, the body detoxifies bromide. Higher intake of an unrefined salt can provide chloride to ease this detoxification.

It's also important to note that iodine works with selenium. 1-3 Brazil nuts daily or the safer supplemental form of selenium (methylselenocysteine) can be taken at 100-200mcg a day.

Since all minerals work together, and too much of any mineral can be detrimental, this is why I recommend a mineral test to find your specific needs through spectracell.com

Coconut oil also supports the thyroid function and taking 1-3 tablespoons a day will provide the thyroid with nourishment.

If you're worried about the health of your thyroid, please seek the professional care of an integrative physician. You can find a physician through acam.org or ICIM.

37: Top 5 Supplements On A Budget

Being someone that studies health, nutrition, and the countless variety of new innovations in supplements, I've found it can be easy to get overwhelmed with all of the recommendations and options out there for supplementation.

I should note the most important thing is to eat a good diet to get most of your nutrients. One bonus tip to enhance the nutrients you absorb from food is to use digestive enyzmes. I personally have used and like Twinlab's Digestive Enzyme blend at www.amazon.com/Twinlab-Enzyme-Maximum-Strength-Capsules/dp/B000GCAVH4 and have found it to be effective.

I also believe **raw** apple cider vinegar is practically a *must use* product for its ability to aid in digestion, prevent heartburn, and provide beneficial enzymes at 1 teaspoon - 1 tablespoon diluted in water with meals. This could be a tip all unto itself going on about its benefits, but I decided to simply insert it here as it can provide missing nutrients and help absorb more nutrients from the diet. It doesn't matter how great your diet is if you aren't properly digesting and absorbing the food you eat.

I'll also note once again that GlutImmune and N-Aceytl Glucosamine can repair gut damage which is another cause of poor nutrient absorption.

But no matter how great your diet and digestion is, in modern times, a great diet usually isn't enough anymore to offset the unnatural world we live in. If you've read these tips and find yourself overwhelmed with options for things to take, don't worry. I've spent the money and done the research for you to bring you my top picks for maximizing your health and longevity without costing a fortune.

Here are what I consider to be the best supplements for the money:

- Vitamin D3 – An incredibly common deficiency that can be readily fixed. Very affordable at less than $2 a month at high doses.

- Ashwagandha – Adaptogenic herb that fights stress and balances adrenals and thyroid. Sensoril extract provides effective dose at $3 a month. Affordable Alternative: Dragon Herbs Longevity Tea from dragonherbs.com.

- Astaxanthin – The most powerful and safe antioxidant (protects against aging and cell damage) I've studied. Crosses the blood brain barrier to protect the brain, protects the skin from UV damage, aids in exercise recovery, reduces excess inflammation, and effective at 4mg a day doses which is around $6-7 a month.

- Fish Oil – A large container of fish oil will provide much needed Omega 3s for a few dollars a month (depending on source) at 3-5 grams a day.

- Organic Powder Spirulina (or Greens Formula) – Provides phytonutrients, chlorophyll, trace minerals, vitamins, healthy fats, and numerous health benefits. Approximately $10 a month for a 5 gram a day dosage. Alternatives: Broken cell wall chlorella, Vitamineral Green by HealthForce, or Moringa powder.

Prices based on amazon.com prices through brands found here: excuseproof.com/favorite-supplements.

These 5 supplements will address the major deficiencies and needs that the typical person will have for around for around $25 a month, or a little less than $1 a day for better health. They'll provide vitamins and minerals in whole food form rather than synthetic form, provide essential fats, combat excess inflammation which is at the root of many degenerate diseases and weight problems, help detoxify the body, and provide on-going anti-aging protection.

While supplements are great, they don't replace the essentials of a healthy diet or completely offset the damage of a poor diet. I suggest including high levels of turmeric as a spice, sea vegetables like kelp and dulse, cultured foods like sauerkraut and kefir, seasonal fruits and vegetables, if consuming animal products getting them from a quality and humane source fed a natural diet, and consider using coconut oil in one's diet to fill in some of the other nutritional deficiencies that are common.

Realize that poor quality food choices, stress, smoking, and even a lot of exercise will quickly deplete the body of essential nutrients that can't always be replaced without heavy supplementation to offset the damage.

38: What Really Works To Detox?

"Detox" has become a buzz word in recent times, but is there any truth to the idea that your body is filled with toxins that need to be removed, or is this just a gimmick to sell high priced "detox" products?

The truth may be somewhere in the middle. The body does quite a good job already of detoxifying the various things it comes into contact with each day, but the problem is our modern day world with stress, poor diets, and man-made toxins that were never found in human history which may push the body beyond what it is capable of handling without some support. All anything can do however is support the body's natural detoxification mechanisms.

One thing to understand is that the body often stores away toxins such as pesticides in fat cells to prevent damage to the rest of the body. A person may feel fine for years as their intelligent body keeps these toxins tucked away, but if they suddenly lose a lot of fat, they may experience sickness associated with toxins being released back into the blood stream from the fat cells. It's then very important that these toxins are properly removed from the body so they don't get reabsorbed.

There is also the issue of parasites which, despite the thinking that they only occur in third world countries, are likely a regular presence in many people even if one doesn't experience overt symptoms.

Add to this the increase in radition exposure, heavy metals in foods, and poor air quality, and you've got a pretty significant need to give the body some extra firepower to handle these toxins.

Let's take a look at the simplest things you can do to keep your body squeaky clean. This is far from everything there is out there, but it's what I consider to be the safest and most practical.

- **Water** – The most important thing you can ingest is a lot of pure water. While coffee and tea are fine, realize they don't have the same effect as pure water and are not a replacement. And 8 glasses a day is rarely enough for a physically active person. I typically drink around a gallon a day, but you should base your water needs on making sure your urine is a light yellow and not allowing yourself to get very thirsty. The proper amount varies for everyone depending on their circumstances. But just drinking water isn't enough, it should be the right kind of water. The ideal water to drink is spring water, although distilled water and reverse osmosis water is fine. Contrary to what some have said, I've found no evidence that distilled water "leaches" minerals. But if you'd like to be safe, simply add some fresh squeezed lemon to the water. Tap water, while sterile, is often filled with chlorine, heavy metals and fluoride. While likely not an issue on occasion, I consider getting a high quality water to be of the utmost important. Avoid exposing water in plastic containers to high heat and preferably store in glass when possible.

- **Clay** – Eating clay is a common occurrence among tribal people, and it may be because they instinctively know that clays like bentonite clay are powerful at removing toxins (which are found even in natural whole foods) from the body. Bentonite or terramin clay has a strong negative charge which pulls toxins from around the body into the intestines where it then binds to the clay to be safely removed. These clays are so strong, they've been shown to be effective at removing radioactive isotopes from the body. Clays can also be used in a bath to draw out toxins from the skin. HealthForce makes an effective clay formula called ZeoForce. 1 - 3 tablespoons daily.

- **Zeolites, Activated Charcoal, Humic and Fulvic Acid** – Zeolites, activated charcoal, and humic/fulvic acids work similar to clay in that they draw toxins to them to bind and safely remove from the body. You can often find formulas with a variety of these ingredients designed to effectively detoxify the body. They're all effective and recommended. Dr. Laszlo's Metal Shield available from Swanson Vitamins is an affordable source of Humifulvate (Humic and Fulvic acid) available at swansonvitamins.com/swanson-ultra-dr-laszlo-meszaros-metal-shield-30-caps.

- **Parasite Cleansers** – To effectively fight parasites, the most common formulas utilize wormfood, cloves, and black walnut hull which takes care of them in all of their life cycles. Food grade diatomaceous earth is an inexpensive way to also kill parasites without hurting healthy cells in both humans and animals. Finally, eating raw garlic is effective at killing parasites.

- **Far Infrared Sauna** – Saunas, and in particular far infrared saunas, are able to draw out toxins through the skin through sweating while providing cardiovascular benefits.

- **Calcium D-Glucarate** – Calcium D-Glucarate is a naturally occurring substance found in fruits and vegetables that is effective at detoxifying a number of things, but is particularly recommended for ridding the body of hormone build up such as excess estrogen which is an issue for both men and women. It may be effective at protecting against cancer. Dosage is 1500 - 3000 mg daily. More information at www.thorne.com/altmedrev/.fulltext/7/4/336.pdf.

- **Diindolylmethane (DIM) and Indole-3-Carbinol (I3C)** – DIM and I3C are compounds found in cruciferous vegetables like broccoli and cauliflower that help reduce levels of "bad" estrogens and increase levels of "good" estrogen making them a good complement to Calcium D-Glucarate. These are very powerful compounds that may be the reason why cruciferous vegetables are so cancer protective. They can also have benefits for enhancing fertility, improving mood, and promoting total hormone balance. There is some debate as to which one is better. I suggest 150-300mg daily of Bioresponse DIM as I've found more research to support it, but both DIM and I3C may be taken in a formula. As a bonus tip for women suffering from cellulite, DIM and Calcium D-Glucarate may be beneficial for reducing cellulite (and acne in both sexes) related to estrogen and hormone imbalance.

- **Trimethylglycine (TMG) and Methyl Donors** – Certain nutrients are what are considered "methyl donors" and they're found in many of the whole foods we eat. These can have a beneficial impact on epigenetic expression. Rather than go into detail here, check out this article which summarizes a lot of important aspects of methyl donors: learn.genetics.utah.edu/content/epigenetics/nutrition Supplementing with a methyl donor like TMG (also called betaine and is found is beets) as well as eating methyl rich foods like cruciferous vegetables and beets provides the body what it needs to properly detoxify itself.

39: Sports Supplements That Aren't Just Hype

The fitness supplement world is filled with promises of getting your dream body virtually overnight by just popping a few high priced pills. Whether it's losing 30 pounds of fat in 30 days, gaining 30 pounds of muscle in 30 days, or adding 30 pounds to one's bench press in 30 days, there's a pill that promises to do it all.

With all the ads and hype, it's no wonder I hear so many people asking me about XYZ supplement to burn fat or gain muscle and strength. As much as I think supplements can be useful, in my nine years of trying almost everything under the sun, I can say pretty confidently that the vast majority of these supplements don't live up to their hype. Many don't work, and the ones that do work aren't worth the money.

But every now and then there's something that comes along that is totally worth the money. Here are my favorite supplement recommendations for fat loss and fitness.

Fat Loss:

- Caffeine – While I don't typically recommend people go crazy with stimulants, there is no doubt that caffeine works for suppressing appetite and enhancing fat loss. I recommend coffee and tea over synthetic caffeine pills, but either way works. My biggest issue here would be to be careful with supplements that contain a lot of caffeine. A couple cups of coffee or tea is cheaper and safer, and some over the counter fat burners/energy drinks can be dangerous leading to worn out adrenal glands.

- Green Tea Extract – This isn't a miracle cure for burning fat, but then again, few supplements are. I recommend green tea extract due to its other health benefits along with its fat burning effects.

- MCT Oil – Already addressed this early, but I'll repeat that this is a safe and simple way to promote fat burning as well as provide a good source of energy.

- Caralluma – Caralluma is a cactus that offers similar appetite suppressing qualities as hoodia, but without all the hype surrounding it even though it may be more effective. It promotes appetite suppression and fat loss while preserving muscle. Caralluma can be purchased from dragonherbs.com

- Yohimbine – Yohimbine is a stimulant that may not be tolerated by some. While I don't recommend the majority of people utilize caffeine or yohimbine (instead utilize adaptogenic herbs) for fat loss, it can be effective at burning fat in trouble spots. Certain areas of the body, like the hips and thighs on women, may be resistant to fat loss while other areas lose fat easily. This is because these trouble spots have higher levels of Alpha 2 Adrenergic receptors which prevent fat oxidation (fat loss) in those areas. Yohimbine is effective at specifically reducing trouble body fat by blocking these Alpha 2 receptors and allowing more fat to be burned from those areas. It is an incredibly common supplement among bodybuilders and figure models who need to reduce stubborn body fat. Dosage is .2mg per kg of bodyweight.

Muscle And Strength:

- Creatine – The most researched and proven sports supplement for enhancing muscle and strength. It will increase water in muscles adding some water weight, but the additional strength will allow many to increase their muscle mass more than normal. 5 grams after a workout is the typical dose, and loading is not necessary. I recommend Creapure creatine for purity.

- Beta Alanine – Beta alanine is not as heavily researched as creatine, but it can be effective for increasing muscle carnosine levels which help resist fatigue. This means more reps done with a given weight potentially increasing muscle mass.

- BCAAs and L-Leucine – Branched chain amino acids are found in significant quantities in protein sources like whey making them somewhat unnecessary for the average person. But I've found benefits from taking additional BCAAs when utilizing very intense training programs to enhance recovery. L-leucine is a particular BCAA that is the signal for muscle growth. Adding in additional BCAAs or leucine (3-5 grams) with meals may help enhance muscle growth when training intensely.

A note on Nitric Oxide and pre-workout supplements: I don't have an issue with any of these things per-se, but I've found them to have minimal impact and not be worth the money. Most of the energy and strength comes simply from the caffeine. The money spent on these high priced supplements can be spent on quality food, adaptogenic herbs, and a greens formulas that will do more to enhance your health (and therefore resistance training efforts) far more than the vast majority of the "muscle-mag" supplements pushed at supplement retailers. Omega Sport's Ultima is my favorite pre-workout formula.

That being said, there are plenty of other effective supplements that may be worth the money depending on your goals. Every now and then I mess around with new herbal formulas and find something I like, but it's rarely worth the high price for the minimal increase of muscle and strength. I suggest not getting caught up in new product hype unless coming from a very reputable company, and giving new products a couple years to see if they stand the test of time.

40: How Not To Get Ripped Off Buying Supplements

Go into a typical supplement retailer, and you can start spending a fortune to get just a few basic supplements like vitamins, protein, and superfood formulas. But over the years, I've developed a nice list of resources for where I could find the highest quality products at a wholesale price.

Here are my best resources for getting quality products at a discount:

- TrueNutrition.com – True Nutrition (formerly True Protein) is my favorite source for picking up protein at wholesale prices. Their hemp protein and pea protein are quality vegan proteins. The top left of their website has the section for their raw ingredients where you can get wholesale protein and custom mix your own protein blends and meal replacements. Use discount code DKD714 to save on your order. Phone at: 760.433.5376

- ProteinFactory.com – Similar to True Nutrition, offers a wide array of various protein and other supplements at affordable wholesale prices. Carries many of the highest quality proteins available anywhere I've seen. Phone: 1.800.343.1803

- iHerb.com – One of the largest selections of health supplements at some of the lowest prices. They also offer free shipping on orders over $40. Use code hec508 to save $5-$10 on your first order.

- NutraPlanet.com – NutraPlanet has very good prices on many brand name sports supplements and they carry their own line of bulk powders and proteins at a much more affordable price than retail. They often has holiday specials for incredible deals far below retail.

- Bodybuilding.com/store – Not always the cheapest, but by far the widest selection and the ability to price-match other advertised prices.

- SwansonVitamins.com – Swanson carries their own line of very high quality supplements of virtually every type. It is often my first stop to find one particular vitamin or herb as they carry quite a selection. They also carry other brands and are the exclusive distributors of a number of health products. Great place to purchase coconut oil at an affordable price. 1.800.824.4491

- LongevityWarehouse.com – A variety of herbs and powders that can't be found anywhere else. My recommended source for quality cacao, moringa, and other health supplements.

41: Dirt Cheap Dumbbells

Even though I work out at a gym, there were times where I found myself unable to go because the gym was closed or I was short on time. This led me to looking into home workouts that I could do to stay strong, and I developed some innovative ways to get in a great workout with just my body weight.

But some muscles, like the back and biceps, are virtually impossible to work without some sort of external equipment like weights, a pullup bar, or resistance bands.

Since I didn't want to invest in setting up an entire home gym full of dumbbells and barbells for the occasional home workouts, I utilized a few simple things to work these muscles such as using a pullup bar, gymnastic rings, a rope to climb, resistance bands, and the thing I'm about to reveal to you now – dirt cheap dumbbells.

Dirt cheap dumbbells are found many stores, but for some reason they don't stick them in the sporting goods section. They're actually more common in grocery stores than anywhere else.

These "dumbbells" are nothing more than the 1-5 gallon water containers/jugs. They range in price from $1-$7, they're adjustable in weight, and they offer a unique type of resistance that really challenges the muscles due to the moving of the water. I like to find the kind that have handles that are easy to grip and move around. You may have to shop around for a kind that are comfortable for use.

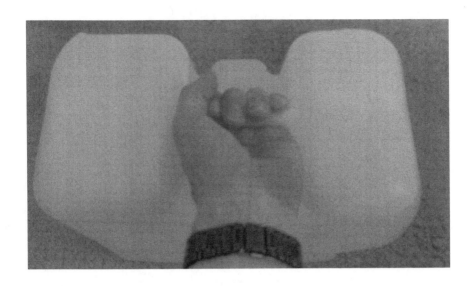

Water jug to weight conversion:

- 1/2 gallon = 4 pounds

- 1 gallon = 8 pounds

- 2 gallons = 16 pounds

- 2.5 gallons = 20 pounds

- 3 gallons = 24

If I had a budget, then just getting a couple 1 and 2.5 gallon water containers would be all I need to get in a good workout. For the smaller containers, I'll usually drink the water, then replace it with tap water for use as a weight. For larger jugs, I use my "stockpile" water that I have for emergencies so I'm actually not spending "extra" money to get these.

Great exercises for water jug dumbbells are (simply swap out water jugs for dumbbells):

Back and Biceps

Water Jug Rows: http://youtu.be/pYcpY20QaE8

Water Jug Bicep Curls: http://youtu.be/av7-8igSXTs

Use the next two exercises if water jugs aren't enough resistance for rows.

Water Jug Straight Arm Rows: http://youtu.be/LaaVZ7u0x2Y

Water Jug Rear Deltoid Raise: http://youtu.be/mtUE9FSu_Uk

Chest and Triceps

Water Jug Floor Flys: http://youtu.be/f5EMDU6d9fY

Water Jug Overhead Tricep Extensions: http://youtu.be/h1ohswSdVZs

If water jugs are too light for overhead extensions, use kickbacks.

Water Jug Tricep Kickback: http://youtu.be/6SS6K3lAwZ8

Shoulders

Water Jug Shoulder Press: http://youtu.be/B-aVuyhvLHU

Use Y shoulder press if water jugs are too light for regular shoulder press:

Water Jug Y-Press: http://youtu.be/IKZjf7lCrdQ

Water Jug Lateral Raises: http://youtu.be/geenhiHju-o

Legs

Water Jug Goblet Squat: http://youtu.be/wbZac-6H9bs

Water Jug Lunge: http://youtu.be/D7KaRcUTQeE

Water Jug Step Up: http://youtu.be/-wcgEGQN5_U (Trick to step-ups, lift the toes of the foot on the floor upwards to increase stress on the working leg that is elevated)

42: Ultimate Home Gym On A Budget

Besides utilizing water jug dumbbells, you can set up a home gym that will meet virtually any fitness goals with only a handful of things. These are things I consider basic home gym equipment:

- Doorway Pull-Up Bar: Typically under $30 and useful for upper back exercises as well as for attaching things like gymnastic rings or ab straps.

- Water Jug Dumbbells: 1, 2.5, and/or 3-5 gallon jugs filled with various levels of water.

- Resistance Bands: A good set will include an anchor for attaching to a doorway. They offer a unique type of resistance that can't be duplicated with free weights. They are also portable so you can take them with you on the go and get in a workout anywhere.

- Ab Wheel: Forget about the hyped up infomercial ab products, this is what *really* works and it only costs around $10.

Here are some additional things for a more "hardcore" home gym on a budget.

- Sandbags: Affordable and a unique type of resistance.

- Gymnastic Rings: The **ultimate** way to train the upper body. Attach to a pullup bar or high ceiling.

- Swiss Ball: Useful for a variety of core training exercises. I personally like to use these for doing bodyweight leg curls as hamstrings are more difficult to hit with bodyweight exercises. http://youtu.be/HAZVSFQ7Y2s

- Dumbbells and Barbells: Getting a set of dumbbells, barbells, and a squat rack will essentially give you a true home gym. To find these on a budget, shop around craigslist and local garage sales.

Department stores, ebay, and craigslist may have equipment at a discount.

43: The Best Exercise You're Probably Not Doing

Want to know a form of exercise that is more fun, effective, and easier on the joints than jogging? This is something so effective, NASA used it to train their astronauts. It is something you can even do while watching your favorite TV show!

The exercise is jumping on a trampoline which is referred to as rebounding.

Rebounding very effectively increases total body oxygenation. The g-force produced during the rebounding literally strengthens every cell in the body and aids in detoxification through enhanced lymph flow.

The best part is, with a mini-trampoline, you can do this exercise virtually anywhere. Even in a relatively small room or outside on a nice day. No need for a bulky and expensive treadmill or cardio machine.

I've heard some people say that even though they hate exercise, they've become addicted to rebounding. It can almost take on a meditative quality.

Affordable mini-trampolines are widely available, but the best built and highest quality rebounders are made by Cellerciser.

If you're tired of treadmills and boring cardio machines, now you know how to get better results, faster, with less joint stress and better health benefits by going back to the fun kids enjoy!

44: Cardio Routines For Busy People

I really feel sorry for the people that think they need to spend hours each week slaving away with boring cardio and aerobics routines to enhance endurance and burn fat. Not only are extended cardio sessions not necessary for fat loss, but they're typically not even the most effective way to build endurance and performance.

That's not to say they don't have their place, but for people on a busy schedule, it's all about getting the greatest results in the least amount of time. This means utilizing high intensity efforts done in short bursts like sprints and interval training.

Here are some of my favorite cardio routines for busy people:

- Kettlebell Swings: If you only had 10 minutes to spare *a week* to exercise and could only do one thing, just do these. 10-20 minutes a week is all you need when done right, but it will be intense. Kettlebell swings (or dumbbell swings if you don't have kettlebells) are one of the best exercises for a better butt and more athletic power. Aim for 75 total reps in a session. Rest around 60 seconds between sets. Do this 2-3 times a week. See Tim Ferriss demonstrate how to do them here: http://excuseproof.com/kettlebell

- Speed Walking: Speed walking is a way to condition the body without letting it adapt to the workout. Many aerobics routines lose their effectiveness at burning fat as the body adapts to them, but speed walking is so inefficient (a good thing) that it continually challenges the body each workout. It is also low-impact for those with joint issues. The process is simple, walk as fast as you can for 15-20 minutes. Attempt to beat the distance covered next session. This can be more challenging than jogging when you really push yourself.

- Incline Challenge: Similar to speed walking, set up a treadmill on a high incline and attempt to walk as fast as possible for 15-20 minutes. The incline really works the calves and glutes and makes this especially challenging without stressing the joints as much as running.

- Sprints and High Intensity Interval Training (HIIT): Sprints, including hill sprints, and other forms of high intensity interval training are a great way to condition the body. HIIT is intense, and need to be treated like any other form of intense exercise by getting adequate rest between sessions. A simple routine would be, after warming up, apply all out effort for 30 seconds such as an all out sprint or cycle. Then drop back to low intensity effort such as walking or slow cycling for 1:30. Repeat this for 4-6 total cycles done at most 3 times a week.

- Multi-Tasking: It may seem obvious, but not everyone thinks to take walk during a phone call or while listening to an audio book. Even if it's just pacing around an office or room during a phone call set to speaker phone, this is a way to do something you'd normally be doing (talking on the phone) but adding in physical activity at the same time. Other examples could be biking to work while listening to an audio book to kill three birds with one stone. Get creative and you may be surprised to find there's a lot of "extra" time you have during the day to be physically active.

45: How To Cut Resistance Training Time In Half

Generally speaking, I recommend following set training routines that are adapted to a person's specific goals and not messing with them. The reason is that if these routines were designed by an intelligent trainer, there's likely a reason everything is laid out as it is.

Nevertheless, sometimes there are some routines that are structured in a way that completely waste time that could be better utilized. That time is the time spent resting between sets.

When analyzing many resistance training routines, you'll see that more often than not the majority of the time is spent resting. In fact, some high intensity routines may only have you doing a few minutes of actual lifting per 30-45 minute workout!

Let's say you have a full body workout routine done three times a week with these exercises:

Squat 3x12

Calf Raises 3x15

Bench Press 3x10

Barbell Rows 3x12

Barbell Curls 3x12

Tricep Pushdowns 3x12

If each set took 1 minute to complete, that means you spend approximately 18 minutes doing actual lifting. If the routine calls for 2 minutes rest between sets, that means you're spending about 2/3 of an almost hour long workout just resting between sets!

We can take this exact same workout and reduce the workout time by around 50%. All we have to do is use supersets/alternating sets. That means going from one exercise to another back and fourth in alternating fashion so two exercises are completed in the time it would normally take to complete one.

Let's look at how we can set up a superset workout using the previous template:

A1. Squat 3x12 – Rest 30 seconds after set, then move onto Calf Raises

A2. Calf Raises 3x15 – Rest 30 seconds after set, then go back to Squats - Repeat cycle until all three sets completed.

B1. Bench Press 3x10 - Rest 30 seconds after set, then move onto Barbell Rows

B2. Barbell Rows 3x12 - Rest 30 seconds after set, then go back to Bench Press - Repeat cycle until all three sets completed.

C1. Barbell Curls 3x12 - Rest 30 seconds after set, then move onto Tricep Pushdowns

C2. Tricep Pushdowns 3x12 - Rest 30 seconds after set, then go back to Barbell Curls - Repeat cycle until all three sets completed.

A side benefit is that the reduced rest time also builds up cardiovascular conditioning.

Another way to utilize supersets is something called "active rest." This means doing "assistance" exercises that aren't very demanding like calf exercises, rotator cuff work, and forearm exercises while resting between sets for your "primary" exercises. This way you can get extra work without adding additional time to your workouts.

For instance, I rarely do ab or calf exercises by themselves. Rather, I do them while "resting" between sets for other exercises.

46: Develop Superhuman Strength

I'm not the strongest guy out there by any means, but being someone who went from getting crushed under a 135 lb barbell trying to max out on bench press shortly after getting into training, to a few years later bench pressing 315 lbs for a set of three (full range of motion and no assistance) at a body weight of 165 pounds as well as completing a full range of motion one arm chinup with ease, I like to think I've picked up a thing or two about maximizing strength.

While I defer most people to seek the help of a qualified strength coach for setting up their training, here are a few tactics that have made a huge difference in maximizing performance that you can start to incorporate easily into your current routine:

- **Utilize Activation Sets**: Activation sets, as opposed to warmup sets, are meant to stimulate the nervous system for a particular exercise without fatiguing the muscle. These activation sets usually call for an extremely explosive movement to amp up the nervous system. An example would be to do a couple high jumps before squatting, or do a single explosive rep on a squat at a relatively heavy weight that doesn't wear the muscles out. My preferred activation exercises are: High jumps before squatting. Explosive pushups (think clapping pushups) off a bench before bench pressing, and explosive pullups before back exercises.

- **Utilize Slow Sets**: While explosive lifts are important for activating the fast twitch muscle fibers, slow sets are important for taking out momentum and working a muscle through the full range of motion. I noticed huge gains in my squat numbers when I started incorporating sets of squats with a 3 second descent, a 3 second pause at the bottom, and a 3 second raise. This strengthened the bottom portion in particular which was my weak link to getting stronger on the lift.

- **Utilize Dead-Start Sets**: A set done from a dead start

means there is no lowering of the weight before it is lifted. Setting up a bench in a squat rack, setting a barbell just above chest level on the pins, and then pressing starting from the bottom portion of the movement is a challenging stimulus that takes the stretch-reflex (momentum) out of the exercise putting tremendous tension on the chest. Utilizing this technique in my training was part of how I was able to work up to a double bodyweight bench press at one point. Pausing for several seconds in the stretched position of a lift is another way to accomplish a similar outcome.

Here's a sample of how I would set up a squat routine to utilize these things:

- 8 reps at 135 to warm up

- 3 high jumps for activation

- 2 super slow reps, then 1 explosive reps at 185 for activation

- 3 explosive reps at 225

- 1 slow rep at 275

- 1 explosive rep at 275

- 1 explosive heavy rep at 305

- Start doing work sets at 315

- After work sets, drop weight down to 225 – 275 and do 1 set with 3-3-3 tempo OR do 1 set from a dead start. Sets are not typically done to absolute failure, but close.

Recommended Strength Training Routines:

Starting Strength:
startingstrength.wikia.com/wiki/The_Starting_Strength_Novice/Beginner_Programs

5/3/1:

t-nation.com/free_online_article/sports_body_training_performance/how_to_build_pure_strength

<u>Westside:</u>

t-nation.com/free_online_article/sports_body_training_performance/westside_for_skinny_bastards

<u>I Bodybuilder:</u>

t-nation.com/free_online_program/sports_body_training_muscle_anaconda/anaconda_protocol#2-8211-training-program/phase-1-8212-shoulders/monday

<u>Gymnastic Bodies:</u> Great resource for building high level strength with body weight and gymnastic workouts at gymnasticbodies.com

47: Anywhere Exercises

What do you do when you don't even have a 20-30 minute block of time to exercise?

The answer is to do a bunch of mini exercise sessions which add up over the course of a day and week. This could mean simply doing a set of pushups during a minute break at work.

But of course this requires knowing which exercises you can do anytime, anywhere. I've found that, with the exception of the back, you can work out most major muscle groups through a full range of motion with a few basic body weight exercises and no equipment.

But even if you can't do these exercises, you can still do a form of isometric resistance exercise anywhere. While not as ideal, isometric exercises can provide a stimulus to the muscles to maintain and increase strength with the benefit of not needing much if any equipment.

Anywhere Leg Exercises:

- Bodyweight Squats http://youtu.be/R1v152b72lo

- Lunges http://youtu.be/rziYBKhDztI

- Step Ups (on chair) http://youtu.be/aaDlSd8rWXY

- Glute Bridge http://youtu.be/uU2xYwNzV4c

- Single Leg Chair Squats http://youtu.be/ftTRZT3rsT8

- Calf Raises http://youtu.be/8OughJl0WAo

- Jumps http://youtu.be/cOFOa4qK34o

- Isometric Deadlift - Find an immovable object, bend down into a semi-squat position and attempt to lift up (like deadlifting) with as much force as possible for 5-10 seconds. One may use a car as an example. http://youtu.be/EC26chZ2b1A

- Wall Squat Holds http://youtu.be/z68npwMKp08

Anywhere Ab Exercises:

- <u>Lying Leg Raises</u> http://youtu.be/1CQg5cyrL3Q

- <u>V-Ups</u> http://youtu.be/CRCprXsWSI4

- <u>Bicycle Crunches</u> http://youtu.be/ixQGJ3Ja-2I

- <u>Planks and Side Planks</u> http://youtu.be/6I990Wbr1JE

- <u>L-Sits</u> http://youtu.be/Y3MxXpaHtaE

Anywhere Pushing Exercises:

- <u>Pushups</u> http://youtu.be/UayvOd0xlAU

- <u>Pushups - Legs Elevated</u> http://youtu.be/2UCEcNuTx8U

- <u>Closer Grip Pushups</u> http://youtu.be/CWkkn0uo-P4

- <u>Pushups – Hands Near Hips</u> http://youtu.be/7f-wV5s3r_Q

- <u>Handstand Pushups</u> http://youtu.be/YdBSefJNbB8

- <u>One Arm Pushups</u> http://youtu.be/UzkDI0_4I2g

- <u>Tuck Planche Pushups</u> http://youtu.be/r1nO8FRtQX8

- <u>Planche Pushups</u> http://youtu.be/oyuJ3T0sQ88

Anywhere Back Exercises (Requires Resistance Bands):

- <u>Resistance Band Pull Aparts</u> http://youtu.be/BVehf-8FAxQ

- <u>Resistance Band Rows</u> http://youtu.be/SLyQL5FVKxU

Self-Resistance Home Workout
- http://youtu.be/kA78Dtu2-q4

48: Six Pack Secrets

One of the biggest questions someone like myself gets is "how do I get a six pack?"

The brutally honest answer is that six pack abs have almost nothing to do with how you train them. It's all about having low body fat which is most commonly a result of the diet. A six pack has very little to do with building, strengthing, or "toning" the abdominals, although those things can help make them pop out a little more. A person can do virtually no direct ab training and still have a ripped six pack as a result of low body fat and the abs being stimulated by other exercises like squats and overhead press.

The next question would be, "how do I get rid of stubborn stomach fat?"

The answer, once again, is a good diet. But the caveat here is that if a person is lean everywhere else but they store stubborn fat on the stomach, it may be a sign of excess cortisol. This is taken care of by the stress reduction tips provided earlier in the guide as well as my recommendation for Ashwagandha and getting grounded through an earthing mat (earthing.com).

While it's possible that direct abdominal training could lead to increased blood flow to the abdominal area and potentially result in some minor spot reduction (which may not totally be a myth), I wouldn't bank on this making all that much of a difference.

Even though many people are overstressed, chances are if a person has too much belly fat, it likely is just a matter of them not being lean enough in general. It takes being very lean to have a visible six pack. And people sometimes kid themselves when estimating their body fat percentage.

With that out of the way, are there better or worse ways to train the abs for improved performance and appearance?

Of course, and it starts with dropping all the countless crunches and sit-ups. A) They're not going to get you a six pack and B) there are better exercises for the abs.

It also means understanding that your abs work to stabilize your torso more than they function to move it. Also, the abdominals often work with the glutes, hip flexors, and lower back to provide optimal core functioning. Strengthening the abs while neglecting the glutes for instance is not a wise idea.

Here are my top picks for the best ab and core exercises:

- Planks and Side Planks: http://youtu.be/6I990Wbr1JE

- Lying Leg Raises: Tip: Keep your lower back pushed into the ground or mat to increase tension on the abs. http://youtu.be/xqTh6NqbAtM

- Hanging Leg Raises: http://youtu.be/hdng3Nm1x_E

- Bird Dog: http://youtu.be/L1kranTPgxI

- Ab Wheel Rollouts: http://youtu.be/HcZG9NqH7SE

49: The Truth About Stretching

Having worked out in a variety of commercial gyms over the years, I see people making all kinds of mistakes with their warm up without them even realizing it. Many times people may be setting themselves up for *increased* chances of injuries and *decreased* performance by simply doing what we've all been told to do – stretching before exercising.

Static stretching, the kind of stretch that's done where a person forces their muscles into a stretched position and holds it there, is generally counter productive when done before a workout for the target muscle group.

Instead, dynamic stretches like arm and leg swings are generally better before a workout, and other forms of stretches are best done on a need-to-do basis after training or on their own.

Yoga or a stretching routine for a specific sport like martial arts are fine on their own, but realize that stretching should be done on a need-to-do basis based on an individual's needs. Getting a particular muscle too limber when it actually needs to be tighter for instance would increase the chance of injury.

Also, forcing the body to stretch beyond where it's comfortable, such as sticking a barbell on someone's back and making them squat as deep as possible even if it's beyond what their body is comfortable doing, can lead to injuries.

The body is smart, and if it's limiting a range of motion, there's usually a good reason for it. So if you find there's an exercise you simply lack the range of motion to do properly – don't do it!

Here's a good article on dynamic warm ups that are better than traditional static stretches:

www.builtlean.com/2011/04/06/dynamic-stretching-routine-best-full-body-warm-up

I have personally used and like Elastic Steel stretching dvds at elasticsteel.net which are targeted towards martial artists, but good for anyone wanting to increase flexibility.

50: How To Not Be A Gym Idiot

Some people have been a gym idiot (myself included) without even realizing it. Remember, awareness is the first step in making a change and I'm here to "aware you" of these cardinal sins of gym etiquette so you never have to worry about committing them.

I'm sure some people disagree with me on a few of these, that's ok. I can't force anyone to be right.

1. **No Curls In The Squat Rack** – A curl can be done with any barbell in the gym, a squat can only be done in the squat rack. This is the greatest gym offense one can commit.

2. **No Blocking The Dumbbell Rack** – All it takes is a few steps back to allow others to access the dumbbell rack. When a person does their exercise right in front of the rack, it blocks access for everyone else the entire time that person does their set.

3. **Put The Weights Back** – I see this gym sin committed more often than any other. Not only is it not very nice to make old ladies have to remove 45 pound plates, but how is anyone supposed to know when someone is done with a piece of equipment if they leave the weights on? I can't tell you how many hours of my life have been wasted from standing around wondering if someone is done with a bench press or squat rack because they left the weights on.

4. **Interrupting Someone During Their Set** – While it's perfectly ok to talk to other people and be sociable in the gym, right in the middle of someone's set is **not** a good time. One should wait until they're finished and see if they have a spare moment. Some people come to train and not chat, so if they don't have time to talk, it's not something to be taken personally.

5. **No Curls In The Squat Rack** – In case someone didn't get the message the first time.

On another note, I'd like to say, particularly to women, to not fear the gym and realize it's generally a welcoming and friendly place.

There are some "women only" or "overweight people only" or "no bodybuilder" type gyms out there that cater to people's fear of the typical commercial gym. While I guess those places are better than nothing (debateable), I want to say most people generally are *not* judging others working out in the gym. Some people are self-conscious about working out in front of others, but realize that many other people there are too busy being self-conscious themselves to give any thought to what others are doing.

If this is an issue, you can ask yourself, "do I want to let the opinions of others stop me from reaching my goals, or would I rather be free to do what's best for me?"

Helpful Resources

Looking for more health and fitness tips:

Besides the resources I've provided in this book, you'll want to check out my free blog, youtube channel, and newsletter with more tips and tricks at:

- excuseproof.com
- youtube.com/excuseproof
- twitter.com/excuseproof
- facebook.com/excuseproof

Also check out my other book "How To Stick To A Diet" for in-depth motivational tips that takes many of the tips here and goes much deeper at: amazon.com/How-Stick-Diet-Unstoppable-ebook/dp/B009GQ4E4W. Since there is some carryover between "How To Stick To A Diet" and this book, if you've purchase both, send me an email at info@excuseproof.com with proof of purchase. I'll send you a special set of bonus mp3s (20 hours of information) with many of my best tips. This is my way of saying thank you for the on-going support and making sure you get 10x your money's worth on anything you purchase from me.

Looking for a specific exercise and diet program for fat loss, health, and/or muscle gain?

There's a lot of hyped up products out there when it comes to diets and exercise programs promising to get people to burn fat and get a "six pack." That being said, there are a few courses I can highly recommend.

My most strongly recommended body transformation program is LGN365 by fitness trainer and author JC Deen of jcdfitness.com.

I had the honor of contributing to this course because I believe in JC's work and the results he gets so much. Read my review of it here: excuseproof.com/lgn365review

I also love Dave Ruel's cookbooks. He has both muscle building and fat burning cookbooks, although realistically you can pretty much use either one for each goal and adjust the serving sizes accordingly. You can find out more at these links:

Fat Loss Recipes: excuseproof.com/fatloss-cookbook

Muscle Gain Recipes: excuseproof.com/muscle-cookbook

Conclusion

Congratulations!

You've made it through the book, great job! You've already shown your commitment to learn. But remember, true knowledge is *applied* knowledge. So get out here and make use of this life changing information. If you have any questions, please contact me at info@excuseproof.com and I will be glad to assist.

With this book, I wanted to create something that was worth at least 10x as much as I charged for it.

So what's my motivation? What do I want?

I want you apply it, change your life, and pay it forward by helping others.

The first way you can pay it forward is by writing a review of this book on amazon.com to let others know of the benefits you've got from it. This will not only help others reach their health and fitness goals by learning these same valuable tips, but it is incredibly rewarding for me to know how much work has benefited you. If there's something I could have done better, let me know that as well so I know how to better serve your needs and the needs of others in reaching their goals.

Thank you!

19815524R00079

Made in the USA
Middletown, DE
05 May 2015